190 Weight Loss Hacks

How to lose weight naturally and permanently without stress

Jane Thurnell-Read

LWB

LIFEWORK
BOOKS

LifeWork Books

1 Brunel View, Exminster

Exeter, England EX6 8FH

Copyright © 2023 by Jane Thurnell-Read

ISBN 978-1-7392941-0-6

Disclaimer

The information in this book is not a substitute for professional advice from your physician or other qualified healthcare provider. If appropriate, please consult with your own physician or healthcare specialist regarding the suggestions and recommendations made in this book.

Do not disregard professional medical advice or delay in seeking it because of something you have read in this book.

This book is not intended for use by people with eating disorders, unless advised to read it by their healthcare provider.

How to eat healthily

Get some free help.

Healthy eating is important whether you're trying to make positive lifestyle changes, negotiate your way through the menopause, lose weight or thrive as you get older. But wanting to eat more healthily doesn't mean it will happen.

Do you often feel like healthy eating demands endless willpower? Does maintaining a balanced diet seem like a constant struggle that overshadows your enjoyment of life?

Imagine how your life would be if you didn't have to guard your eating habits vigilantly.

With my free eBook, **"You Don't Need Willpower to Eat Healthily"**, you'll discover a fresh perspective on healthy eating. This 28-page guide is packed with clear explanations, enlightening insights, and practical worksheets that you can either download or complete online without any hassle.

Regain control of your eating habits with ease.

Download your free copy now and embark on a path to effortless, stress-free healthy eating:

https://www.janethurnellread.com/willpower/

Contents

How To Use This Book

My heart goes out to you if you've tried repeatedly to lose weight without succeeding. I feel for you if you've lost a lot of weight and put it all back on again. You may feel ashamed of yourself for being weak-willed. You may know other people judge you harshly and feel angry that they do. You may feel bewildered that you can be successful in so many areas of your life, but not in this one. Maybe every day is a battle between you and food.

It's simple, right? Eat fewer calories than you use, and you lose weight. So, why can't you do it?

Sadly, in the press, in books and on the web, there has been an emphasis on calorie counting and miracle pills. But slowly other possibilities are being researched. This book gives you 190 hacks to help you lose weight and keep it off for good. It gives you ways to minimise the conflict or hopelessness you may feel.

My original intention had been to write 200 hacks. At one point as I was writing the book, I actually had 216! But I had made a commitment to myself that I wouldn't include "fluff" – hacks that have endlessly been repeated on the web until they appear to be self-evidently true, but they don't have any research to back them up. So, I was ruthless and cut those out. I've ended up with 190 hacks that I'm proud to share with you.

So, how to use this book?

There isn't one best way, although I hope that eventually you will read the whole book. How you use the book initially depends on where you are in your weight control journey.

If you want some quick hacks that you can read and apply quickly, check out Hack 28, Hack 58 and Hack 92. Sometimes small things can make a difference. They may not make a big difference, but over time even small differences mount up. Some of these hacks are almost effortless.

If you're interested in knowing what the research says about low fat diets, high protein diets or high fibre diets check out Hacks 100, 101 and 103.

Do you want to focus on something other than calories, carbohydrates and fat? Check out Hack 37 or Hack 41.

Do you do fine for a while and then get overwhelming cravings? Take a look at Hacks 29, 32, 87 and 88.

Do you feel surrounded by unhelpful people and need some help dealing with them? Check out hacks 57, 132, 138, 147 and 165.

Do you think you need help from a therapist? Check out Hacks 122 to 129 to see what might be helpful for you.

Do you feel a need to reset your whole life? Take a look at Hack 41 and 43.

Do you feel your emotions wreak havoc with your plans, or that pesky negative voice in your head sabotages your best intentions? Check out Hacks 40, 96, 143, and 188.

Do you despair of being able to maintain your weight loss? Are upcoming holidays a nightmare? Check out hacks 70, 71, 107, 162 and 163.

My personal favourite hacks are 01, 08, 31 and 52 and 62.

There are hacks in this book that are appropriate for wherever you are in your relationship with your body and weight management. You obviously can't try everything at once. Find a couple of hacks that speak to you and start with them.

Jane Thurnell-Read

01: Is Willpower & Self-Control Limited?

S tudies in the 1990's showed that our willpower decreases through the day. We have to exert willpower more and more times through the day, but eventually run out. We only have a certain amount of willpower or self-control available.

This idea is used to explain and justify snacking in the evening:

"I've managed all day to restrain myself, but I've now run out of willpower and can't do it anymore. That's just how the brain works, so you can't expect me not to snack in the evening."

Or maybe:

"I've been good all week, so it's only natural I want to pig out over the weekend. I've just run out of willpower, as you'd expect."

Some researchers[1] have attempted to replicate the original research without success. While there are more than 200 studies that show doing a task requiring impulse control and mental effort can lead to a drop in self-control when switching to an unrelated task, it's usually been tested in a laboratory setting.

More recent research[2] in the *European Journal of Personality* has shown that people may be vulnerable to changes in self-control through the day, depending on whether they believe willpower is more or less limited. Limited willpower beliefs might be associated with steeper decreases in self-control across the day, which may result in less goal-consistent behaviour by the evening. Put simply, if you believe willpower is limited, it is!

You may be thinking that you've never thought about willpower being limited, but you do seem to have less of it in the evening. It might be true that you have a harder time controlling what you eat when they are tired at the end of the day, but that doesn't mean that self-control is a limited resource.

Believing that willpower and self-control are limited is likely to get in the way of controlling what you eat.

Understanding that you are likely to make poorer decisions when you are tired, is something you can address.

Associate professor Kathleen Martin Ginis[3], McMaster University (Canada) says:

"There are strategies to help people rejuvenate after their self-regulation is depleted. Listening to music can help; and we also found that if you make specific plans to exercise—in other words, making a commitment to go for a walk at 7 p.m. every evening—then that had a high rate of success."

Jumana Yahya in the academic journal *Frontiers in Psychology*[4] looks at whether self-control solely resides in the brain. She concludes that self-control can be triggered by outside sources. She discusses fist clenching – see Hack 04 - a calm environment and social support as "situated causes". She writes:

"One major practical benefit of unburdening the brain of sole causal responsibility for successful self-control is that exercising this ability becomes exponentially easier. Since situated causes operate non-consciously and in a reflexive-like way, the result can be achieved without conscious effort, and not having to intentionally invest conscious effort greatly reduces – if not eliminates altogether – feelings of struggle or difficulty. Delegating the work of regulating oneself to non-conscious processes thus creates an "effortless" experience. Since the anticipation of struggle or difficulty is what causes many people who face a self-control dilemma to feel too overwhelmed to attempt being self-controlled, a less effortful experience can circumvent this consequence."

Many of the hacks in this book are "situated causes", taking the heavy lifting away from your brain and putting it in the environment. This allows you to create an environment that supports and triggers your efforts at self-control.

O2: Imagine More To Eat Less

We often think we shouldn't obsess about food. We try to distract ourselves, but a study by Carey Morewedge[5] of Carnegie Mellon University (USA), published in *Science*, shows that when you imagine eating a certain food, it reduces your actual consumption of that food.

So, if you're going to a party, imagine as vividly as you can eating the food that is likely to be the big temptation there.

Do you always reach for a salty or sweet snack when you arrive home from work? On the way home imagine as clearly as you can eating and enjoying that snack.

These research findings suggest that trying to suppress your thoughts of desired foods to curb cravings for those foods is a fundamentally flawed strategy. (Also see Hack 03).)

O3: Don't Think About Chocolate!

A necdotally you probably know that if you're told not to think about something, it becomes almost impossible not to think about that thing. That's OK, if I say to you: "Don't think about pink elephants." You may waste some time thinking about pink elephants, but it won't affect how healthy your life is, or what happens to your weight.

But what if you tell yourself not to think about chocolate (or whatever your vice food of choice is)? It then becomes much more difficult to avoid eating it.

D M Wegner[6] and colleagues report on some experiments they conducted on thought suppression in the *Journal Of Personality And Social Psychology*:

"In a first experiment, subjects verbalizing the stream of consciousness for a 5-min period were asked to try not to think of a white bear, but to ring a bell in case they did. As indicated both by mentions and by bell rings, they were unable to suppress the thought as instructed. On being asked after this suppression task to think about the white bear for a 5-min period, these subjects showed significantly more tokens of thought about the bear than did subjects who were asked to think about a white bear from the outset. These observations suggest that attempted thought suppression has paradoxical effects as a self-control strategy, perhaps even producing the very obsession or preoccupation that it is directed against."

So, that's the paradox: being determined not to think about something, means you are more likely to think about that thing.

If you decide not to think about the food/drink you really like, but want to reduce or avoid completely, you are more likely to think about it in an unhealthy way – the forbidden temptation. The last hack showed us anyway that deliberately and purposefully thinking about something high-calorie, means you are likely to eat less of it anyway.

04: Increasing Your Self Control

A study in the *Journal of Consumer Research*[7] says firming your muscles can increase your self-control.

It may seem bizarre but clenching your muscles - any muscles - can help you exert self-control. The next time you feel your willpower slipping as you walk past a fast-food shop, tighten your muscles. You could flex your biceps or tighten your tummy muscles or make a fist.

If you're in a restaurant checking out the menu, squeeze your legs together. (Don't do this while walking past the fast-food place or you might fall over!)

O5: Keep It Simple

This is a simple rule that works for a lot of people. You fill half your plate or bowl with vegetables, fruit or salad and the rest of the plate with whatever you want. The choice is yours.

Professor Brian Wansink[8] says:

"Could a person load up half of their plate with Slim Jims [a US snack food] and bacon? Sure, but they don't. Giving people freedom – a license to eat with only one guideline – seems to keep them in check. There's nothing to rebel against, resist, or work around. As a result, they don't even try. They also don't seem to overeat. They want to eat more pasta and meatballs or another piece of pizza, but if they also have to balance this with a half-plate of fruit, vegetables, or salad, many decide they don't want it bad enough."

Do you like this idea? One simple rule for you to follow. It's not complicated, and it's been shown to work.

Cognitive scientists[9] from Indiana University (USA) and the Max Planck Institute for Human Development in Berlin compared the dieting behaviour of women following two radically different diet plans. They found that the more complicated people thought their diet plan was, the sooner they were likely to drop it.

Peter Todd, professor in Indiana University's Department of Psychological and Brain Sciences said:

"For people on a more complex diet that involves keeping track of quantities and items eaten, their subjective impression of the difficulty of the diet can lead them to give up on it."

Check out Hack 104 on fibre for another simple intervention that can really make a difference.

O6: HALT

D o you find yourself eating without thinking? Do you sometimes just push handfuls of food into your mouth and swallow without tasting. Then HALT may be just what you need.

HALT stands for

- Hungry

- Angry

- Lonely

- Tired

Malia Frey[10], a certified health coach and weight loss expert, says:

"If you frequently find yourself overeating certain foods, consider taking a minute before each eating occasion to examine your physical and emotional needs. Ask yourself a few questions to find out if eating is what your body actually needs in that moment. In many cases, food will not eliminate your discomfort—sometimes, eating may add to it."

Use the acronym HALT to take the time to stop and consider whether you want food because you're hungry or reaching for it for some other reason.

Hilton Head Health[11] says:

"Remember: hunger signals a biological need for nutritious, healthy food to feed our bodies so that we can get energy. Food is fuel, not a panacea for other feelings. Next time we find ourselves eating outside of a normal mealtime, HALT and ask, *am I truly hungry* (stomach growling, been a few hours since I last ate) *or are am I angry, lonely or tired*? We can interrupt the cycle of emotional eating by using HALT to check in with ourselves and honestly address our real needs and feelings."

There are other possibilities. Sometimes you may eat because you're anxious. At other times you may eat out of habit, so maybe you need to use HHAALT!

- Hungry

- Habit

- Angry

- Anxious

- Lonely

- Tired

Whether you use HALT or HHAALT, eating is the correct response only if you are hungry.

Of course, it could be boredom that makes you eat. It could be duty ("I made this for you, please eat it"), but now the acronym is getting complicated. It may be best when you start trying this hack to keep it simple.

Alternatively think what emotions stimulate you to eat when you're not hungry and create your own acronym.

It's been used by professionals to help people who are dealing with addictions, so could be really useful if you feel addicted to food.

O7: Why?

Spend some time thinking about why you've gained weight. Write down all the reasons and opposite them write down your actions to counteract them.

You probably won't complete this all-in-one go. As you think about it, you are likely to go back and want to write more. You may want to add more reasons why, and also add more changes you can make, particularly as you read more of this book!

Remember that there are no right answers. Just write from your heart and see where it takes you.

If you find yourself continually blaming someone else, ask yourself why you let them have this power over you?

If you find you've made the same mistake repeatedly in the past, what can you do now to ensure that doesn't happen again?

08: The Variety Effect

Having a large variety of a particular category of food can mean that you eat more of that food.

So, if you want to reduce your snack intake, reduce the number of different snacks you have available. For example, have either crisps/chips or nuts, but not both. Have one type of biscuits/cookies, not a variety. Have just one flavour of icecream, not a variety.

Limiting your options can mean you eat less. Buy only a limited variety of snacks and treats. That way you may open the fridge or cupboard door and not want to eat anything that's there.

You may feel all the options boring. You may still end up eating something, but there is a chance you'll just sigh and shut the door.

Laura Wilkinson[12], lecturer in Psychology, Swansea University, Wales writes:

"... we asked two groups of volunteers to decorate Christmas trees and gave them chocolates to snack on. We found that, in line with other scientific studies, people will eat more from a bowl containing a variety of flavoured chocolates than a bowl containing only one type of chocolate.

"The "variety effect" is thought to be the result of a phenomenon called "sensory specific satiety". This is where our desire to consume a food of a particular flavour, colour and texture, decreases while we are eating it. This is one of the processes that helps us to stop eating and finish our meal. But this doesn't affect how much we appreciate other foods – and our desire to eat other different foods does not reduce.

"In this way, switching between foods with different flavours interrupts and delays this decline in desire to eat from kicking in. And after a number of interruptions, the meal or snack time becomes longer, and more is eaten overall."

But the variety effect can work for you in another way too. Ms Wilkinson goes on to say:

"This "variety effect" has the potential to be very helpful if you are trying to eat more of a particular food – such as fruits and vegetables"

In other words, have more variety available for foods you want to eat more of and less variety for the things you want to eat less of.

O9: Beware Of Boredom!

A study[13] in the *Journal of Health Psychology* by Amanda C Crockett and colleagues found that boredom may be an important contributor to overeating. You probably already know that you are likely to eat more when you're bored.

So, think now about what you can do next time you're bored. What is the alternative to reaching for that snack? Do you need to make changes in your life if you are often bored?

Both the last hack and this one are about boredom. At first sight, they may seem like opposite conclusions. But the source of the boredom is different.

In the last hack it was the food that was boring. In this hack it's some aspect of your life that is the source of the boredom. What can you do about the boredom in your life?

The Heart Research Institute UK[14] says:

"Find a 'hands-on' activity or hobby that you enjoy. When you keep your hands busy, you can only do one activity at a time – your hands will be too busy to be reaching for food. Activities such as surfing the web, watching TV or reading don't keep your hands busy, and you may be more tempted to eat at the same time. Instead, do a cross-stitch, play an instrument, tinker in the garage, garden, paint, clean ..."

10: Public Weight Goals Public?

Many coaches and web articles advise making goals public as a way of increasing your accountability. If you feel more accountable, you are more likely to achieve your goal. This is one of those pieces of advice that seems to make sense. But the evidence doesn't support this approach.

A study published in the *International Journal of Applied Behavioural Economics*[15], analysed data from 364 clients signed up to an online weight management service. In the trial clients voluntarily completed a baseline survey and then were randomly assigned to one of three different groups.

The first group had to nominate a friend or family member to keep track of whether they had met their weight loss commitment.

The second group was offered a refund on their subscription, regardless of whether they met their target weight in coming weeks.

The third group – the comparison group - comprised of clients who continued to pay the monthly fee, so maintained a financial commitment to achieve their weight loss target.

The study measured weight loss outcomes at 12 weeks and found that all participants lost weight on average. The refund group lost 2.4% on average and the comparison group lost on average 2.2% of initial body weight.

The group that was asked to share their goals with friends or family reported the slowest rate of weight loss with an average of 1.1%.

Researcher Dr Manu Savani said:

"The study shows that increased commitment can have a negative outcome and this may be for a number of different reasons. One reason could be that the involvement of friends or family may act as a substitute for the individuals' own accountability and self-monitoring practice away from the digital tools, undermining weight loss efforts.

"Another reason could be that the take up of additional, reputational commitment to achieve already challenging health goals may have created a sense of 'overload' with participants feeling less motivated and less willing to absorb the short-term trade-offs involved in achieving significant weight loss."

This was also confirmed by a study by psychologist Peter Gollwitzer[16] of New York University (USA). Gollwitzer's study wasn't focussing on weight loss. He and his colleagues were looking at study goals for students. We cannot be sure that the outcome would have been the same if the goals had been to do with weight loss, but it seems likely.

In the results of this study and subsequent studies performed on other students, the experimenters found that the students whose intentions were known tended to act less on their intentions than those whose intentions were unknown.

The researchers concluded that telling people what you want to achieve creates a premature sense of completeness. While you feel a sense of pride in letting people know what you intend to do, that pride doesn't motivate you and can in fact hurt you later.

So, the conclusion here is that it may not be a good idea to tell others of your weight loss goals.

11: Have A Quiet Moment

Have you ever talked to people who have got down to their ideal weight, kept the weight off and look and feel great? Almost all of them had a quiet moment before they started. By this, I mean that they stopped thinking about the future and wishing for change.

They stopped beating themselves up for how they were. They accepted what and who they were and in that quiet moment they made a profound decision. They decided to do what they needed to do to live a healthier life.

Does it sound grandiose to say that in that moment they experienced unconditional love for themselves?

Are you saying: "I couldn't do that"? Remember when you give yourself unconditional love you are not saying you are perfect, but you are loving yourself even with your imperfections.

I'm not saying you must do this all the time, but just for a quiet moment while you accept where you are and commit yourself to something better.

12: Motivate Yourself Excruciatingly

Have you been told to reward yourself for your progress and success? Of course, preferably not with chocolate or a Big Mac. Rewarding yourself may well be helpful, but how about trying something slightly different.

Set yourself a goal and a deadline. If you don't achieve it, decide you will donate some money to a group you totally disagree with if you don't achieve your goal.

Think how excruciating it would be to donate to a political party you detest! What about a charity that you think just wastes money? Get the idea? It has to be a donation that would make you feel extremely uncomfortable and want to squirm.

Could that motivate you?

13: Lazy Self

The Heart Research Institute UK[17] says:

"Let your 'motivated self' look after your 'lazy self'… You don't have to be up-beat and motivated all the time – it's just not possible, and that's ok. When you're feeling like cooking or prepping food, make the most of that time and prepare food for those times when you don't have time or find it difficult. Aim to have easy options, leftovers or homemade frozen meals for those times. Set yourself up for success by thinking ahead and making things as easy for yourself as possible for those tougher days."

Rather than trying to galvanise yourself when you're feeling motivated, concentrate on getting the maximum prep out of yourself when you're buzzing.

14: Eating In A Healthy Restaurant

Researchers Chandon and Wansink[18] asked consumers to guess how many calories were in sandwiches from two restaurants. They estimated that sandwiches contain 35% fewer calories when they come from restaurants claiming to be healthy than when they were from restaurants not making this claim.

The researchers found that consumers then chose beverages, side dishes, and desserts containing up to 131% more calories when the main course was positioned as "healthy" compared to when it was not. In this study the "healthy" main course contained 50% more calories than the "unhealthy" one.

Just because a product is organic or from a small independent restaurant or labelled as healthy, it doesn't mean it's automatically low in calories or healthy for you. A big chain may say it has given its menu a healthy makeover, but don't take that at face value. You need to do your research.

It's also important that you don't think eating a healthy main course, means you can eat and drink whatever else you want.

15: Too Much Light?

A study published *in JAMA Internal Medicine*[19] found that women who slept with some artificial light were more likely to gain weight and develop obesity. The light could be from a television that had been left on, a night light, a mobile phone or streetlights.

The participants, all women, were followed for almost 6 years. Their BMI, weight, waist and hip circumference, etc. were taken at the beginning and the end of the study.

The researchers found that women who slept with a light or television on were more likely to be obese at the start of the study. They were also 17% more likely to have gained around 11 pounds (4.9 kg) or more over the follow-up period. The association with light coming from outside the room was more modest. Using a small nightlight wasn't associated with any more weight gain than sleeping with no light.

The authors couldn't rule out all the other factors that might be linked with artificial light at night and weight gain. However, their findings didn't significantly change when they adjusted for age, having an older spouse or children in the home, race, socioeconomic status, where they lived, calories consumed, night-time snacking, physical activity, and sleep length and quality.

Switching off TVs before you sleep is clearly a sound thing to do. If you use a television to help you sleep, try a radio instead.

16: Should You Skip Breakfast?

The UK NHS[20] is convinced you <u>should</u> eat breakfast:

"Skipping breakfast will not help you lose weight. You could miss out on essential nutrients and you may end up snacking more throughout the day because you feel hungry."

The American Psychological Association[21] says:

"Patients often skip breakfast with the thought they are reducing calories or can "save up" calories for later. But skipping meals can slow your metabolism, make you prone to later eating binges, and have a negative effect on your health."

The British Heart Foundation[22] says:

"There's some evidence that eating breakfast is linked to a lower risk of obesity, supporting the theory that it's better to eat earlier than later. But this is not conclusive."

Research published in the *Journal of Clinical Endocrinology & Metabolism*[23] concluded:

"Eating a big breakfast rather than a large dinner may prevent obesity and high blood sugar."

The Mayo Clinic[24] is less sure:

"Some research suggests that regularly eating a healthy breakfast may help you lose excess weight and maintain your weight loss. But other research suggests that skipping breakfast may not be bad for you and may also help with weight control ... More research is needed to understand the connection between breakfast eating habits and weight control."

So, what should you be doing in the meantime? Find what works for you. Do you eat more if you skip breakfast? Do you eat less healthily later in the day if you skip breakfast? Do you find having breakfast sets you up for the day and reduces cravings?

It may well be that eventually research will show there's not one correct answer to this question. As with many other things, it may vary from person to person.

17: Is Snacking Good Or Bad?

S nacking is controversial! Some authorities say that you need to avoid all snacks if you want to lose weight. Other people say you must snack. Yet others say healthy snacking can be a successful part of weight management.

There have been suggestions that snacking can boost metabolism, but this idea has largely been discounted.

Melina Jampolis[25], M.D., is a board-certified physician nutrition specialist, studying nutrition for weight loss and disease prevention. She says:

"I'm a snacker. I don't do well eating big meals. So I do have to eat every few hours. Not to stimulate my metabolism, but to keep my blood sugar and energy levels stable. But that's the reason for it. Equating it to metabolism...is something I wish would go to the wayside."

The Nutrition Source[26] (Harvard T H Chan, USA) says:

"Snacks have been associated with both weight gain and maintaining weight, as well as with a lower or higher diet quality. Although snacks can be a regular and important part of a healthy diet, they can also lead to health problems. What differentiates the two scenarios is one's snacking behavior: what you snack on, why you snack, frequency of snacking, and how snacks fit into your overall eating plan...

"The concept of meal planning can be applied to snacks. Take the time to incorporate snack planning to ensure that snacks work for you, not against you."

The Heart Research Institute UK[27] says:

"Snacking can be either extremely helpful or extremely damaging to your weight loss or healthy lifestyle choices. Snacking well comes down to being organised so you have something healthy on hand when you need it."

Snacking is important to prevent getting too hungry so that you make poor choices at meals. Thinking that it does something to "boost metabolism" is really an incorrect interpretation of the science.

This seems largely to be the current thinking about snacking – it can be helpful, providing you choose healthy snacks and don't overdo it.

Not everyone agrees. Belinda Lennerz[28], M.D., an endocrinologist and nutrition researcher at Boston Children's Hospital believes that snacking can make you hungrier:

" your body doesn't know you only intended to have a bite or two... Your gut and digestive system react as though a big meal is on the way. The resulting drop in blood sugar can shoot your hunger through the roof ... That can leave you wanting more snacks."

What works for you? This seems to be a case of experimenting to find out whether snacking helps or hinders your weight control journey.

18: Snack Wisely

Professor Brian Wansink in his book *Mindless Eating: Why We Eat More Than We Think* offers this advice about snacking:

"Avoid eating directly from the package. People served a snack mix in a bowl ate 134 fewer calories than those eating straight from the bag."

19: Sleep To Lose Weight

S leeping well can help you lose weight. This is not just because while you're sleeping, you're not eating.

Sleep-deprived people tend to eat more than people who are well-rested. Not getting enough sleep can also lead to a disruption of neurotransmitters and hormones.

The Sleep Foundation[29] says:

"The neurotransmitters ghrelin and leptin are thought to be central to appetite. Ghrelin promotes hunger, and leptin contributes to feeling full. The body naturally increases and decreases the levels of these neurotransmitters throughout the day, signaling the need to consume calories.

"A lack of sleep may affect the body's regulation of these neurotransmitters. In one study, men who got 4 hours of sleep had increased ghrelin and decreased leptin compared to those who got 10 hours of sleep. This dysregulation of ghrelin and leptin may lead to increased appetite and diminished feelings of fullness in people who are sleep deprived."

A study by Stephanie M. Greer and colleagues[30] reports that:

"sleep deprivation significantly decreases activity in appetitive evaluation regions within the human frontal cortex and insula cortex during food desirability choices, combined with a converse amplification of activity within the amygdala. Moreover, this bi-directional change in the profile of brain activity is further associated with a significant increase in the desire for weight-gain promoting high-calorie foods following sleep deprivation, the extent of which is predicted by the subjective severity of sleep loss across participants."

In other words, the shorter you are of sleep the more likely you are to crave high-calorie foods.

Dr. Kara Duraccio[31] of Brigham Young University (USA) says:

"It's human nature to think that when we have a long to-do list, sleep should be the first thing to go or the easiest thing to cut out ... We don't recognize that getting enough sleep helps you accomplish your to-do list better."

But how do you get enough sleep? Try the Headspace app[32]. This has lots of different tracks to choose from. Try their Sleepcasts series for every-changing storytelling in a range of soothing voices. The Wind Downs series lead you through meditation and breathing to prepare you for sleep. Sleep Music gives you calming tracks to help you drift off.

If you're in the UK, BBC Sound has a selection of sleep tracks too.

Or try essential oils, which are widely regarded as having beneficial effects on sleep. There is also now some scientific evidence[33] to support this.

- Lavender[34] helps slow heart rate and relaxes muscles.

- Sweet marjoram is calming and helps to slow the mind.

- Chamomile and Sandalwood help to reduce anxiety.

- Ylang Ylang has a soothing effect that alleviates stress.

- Peppermint oil[35] aids sleep, probably through reducing stress.

Put a few drops of oil on your hands and rub your palms together before smelling them or add essential oils to water and spray in your room or on your pillow.

Other possibilities include developing a healthy evening routine: eliminating screen use for a t least an hour before bed, dimming lights as the evening progresses and having a warm bath or shower.

20: What's Your Time?

Y ou may eat late in the evening, either through preference or convenience, but the research in this area may make you think again.

Research published in the academic journal *Nutrients*[36] concluded:

"... later timing of EI [energy intake, i.e. food and drink] and sleep are associated with higher body fat and lower levels of PA [physical activity] in people with overweight and obesity."

Research published in *The American Journal of Clinical Nutrition*[37] looked at the time between breakfast and dinner, the midway point between breakfast and dinner times. The researchers divided the participants into those who ate early (midpoint of before 14.54) and later eaters (after 14.54). Yes, I know it excludes 14.54 itself, but that's what the research says!

At the beginning of the study, which lasted 19 weeks, no differences were observed in energy intake or physical activity levels between early and late eaters. But late eaters had higher BMI, higher concentrations of triglycerides, and lower insulin sensitivity compared with the early eaters.

During the programme late eaters had an average 80gm lower weekly rate of weight loss on average, higher odds of having weight-loss barriers and lower odds of motivation for weight loss compared with early eaters.

The researchers concluded:

"Our results suggest that late eating is associated with cardiometabolic risk factors and reduced efficacy of a weight-loss intervention."

You may well be dismissing the idea of an extra 80 gm weight loss a week. Over time it will mount up. If you've tried many times to lose weight without lasting success, you need to look at hacks that make even a small difference.

So, what is the midpoint between your breakfast time and your dinner time. If it's later than 2.54 pm, is it possible to change it? This is an easy tweak for many people. Of course, it may initially take some planning to get it right.

21: Late Night Munchies

A study published in the journal *Obesity*[38] found that the body's internal clock, the circadian system, increases hunger and cravings for sweet, starchy and salty foods in the evenings. While the urge to consume more in the evening may have helped our ancestors store energy to survive longer in times of food scarcity, in the current environment of high-calorie food, those late-night snacks may result in significant weight gain.

But before you throw up your hands in despair and think that you can't counteract nature, remember that lots of people do avoid eating in the evenings.

Steven Shea[39], Ph.D., director for the Center for Research on Occupational and Environmental Toxicology at Oregon Health & Science University (USA) and senior author on the study.

"Of course, there are many factors that affect weight gain, principally diet and exercise, but the time of eating also has an effect. We found with this study that the internal circadian system also likely plays a role in today's obesity epidemic because it intensifies hunger at night... People who eat a lot in the evening, especially high-calorie foods and beverages, are more likely to be overweight or obese."

Shea goes on to say:

"If you stay up later, during a time when you're hungrier for high-calorie foods, you're more likely to eat during that time ... You then store energy and get less sleep, both of which contribute to weight gain.

"If weight loss is a goal, it's probably better to eat your larger, higher-calorie meals earlier in the day... Knowing how your body operates will help you make better choices.

Going to bed earlier, getting enough sleep and choosing lower-calorie foods rather than higher-calorie foods in the evening can all help with weight loss."

The Academy of Nutrition & Dietetics[40] says:

"Sleep deprivation can impair glucose metabolism and affect hormones linked to hunger, appetite and body weight regulation. When we get too little sleep, we may confuse tiredness for hunger. If you're tempted to keep snacking after a balanced dinner, that may be a sign that your body needs rest. Adults should strive for 7 to 9 hours of sleep every night."

Nutritionist Liz Weinandy[41] of Ohio State University (USA) writes:

"Oftentimes nighttime snacking is habitual and associated with another activity. The most common example I give is eating while watching television. Sometimes it's really hard to break the habit. You may have to stop watching television or change the location where you watch television. If that doesn't work, see if you can eat something healthier so the snacking isn't doing harm to your health."

She goes on to say:

"Sleep is a big one. When I see patients who are doing a lot of eating late at night, that's one of the first things I ask them. If you're not getting enough sleep, it affects the cortisol levels which can affect the hunger hormones. Plus, if you're up until midnight and you've eaten dinner around 6 o'clock, chances are pretty good that within that five hour window, you're going to get hungry again. Go to bed at 10 if you can."

Sleep seems to be one of the keys for a healthy life and is important for weight management too. Rather than trying to restrain your evening eating, plan to go to sleep sooner. Check out Hack 19 if you struggle to sleep well.

22: Another Reason To Chew

C hewing well helps in digestion. We're also told to chew food slowly so that our body has more chance to register fulness.

But chewing more has another benefit. It increases the thermic effect of food consumption. This means that the more you chew the more calories you use for the whole digestive process. This is because more heat is generated. The production of heat in the body because of eating is known as diet-induced thermogenesis (DIT).

Dr. Yuka Hamada[42] and Professor Naoyuki Hayashi from Waseda University, Japan carried out a research study on chewing. The entire study included three trials conducted on different days.

In the control trial, they asked the volunteers to swallow 20-ml liquid test food normally every 30 seconds.

In the second trial, the volunteers kept the same test food in their mouth for 30 seconds without chewing, thereby allowing prolonged tasting before swallowing.

In the third trial, they studied the effect of both chewing and tasting; the volunteers chewed the 20-mL test food for 30 seconds at a frequency of once per second and then swallowed it.

The variables such as hunger and fullness, gas-exchange variables, DIT, and splanchnic circulation [an area of the abdomen] were measured before and after the test-drink consumption.

The liquid food was used because the researchers wanted to establish whether it was something about chewing or the size of the food eaten that affected the thermogenesis.

There was no difference in hunger and fullness scores among the different groups. But Professor Hayashi said:

"We found DIT or energy production increased after consuming a meal, and it increased with the duration of each taste stimulation and the duration of chewing."

He went on to say:

"While the difference in energy expenditure per meal is small, the cumulative effect gathered during multiple meals, taken over every day and 365 days a year, is substantial."

So, this gives you yet one more reason to chew and savour your food.

23: Restless Sleep

Colin Chapman[43], Uppsala University (Sweden) and colleagues found that people who were deprived of one night's sleep purchased more food (in terms of calories and weight) in a mock supermarket on the following day.

Sleep deprivation also led to increased blood levels of ghrelin, a hormone that increases hunger, on the following morning. The researchers found that there was no correlation between individual ghrelin levels and food purchasing. This suggested that other mechanisms may be more responsible for increased purchasing. A likely one is a reduced ability to control impulsive behaviour.

Regardless of why this happened, the takeaway from this is to avoid shopping after a restless night if possible.

If reduced impulse control is responsible, it's likely that this will affect your ability to say no to high-calorie junk food.

Yet more reasons to get a good night's sleep. See Hack 19 for suggestions on how to do this.

24: Use Self-Checkouts

According to a study from IHL Consulting Group[44], impulse purchases among women drop by 32.1% and men by 16.7% when a self-checkout is used instead of a staffed checkout.

When people use self-checkouts, they see fewer products, such as chocolate, candies and snacks, and so are less likely to buy them. Often the wait is shorter, so exposure time is less even for what is there.

You could also use online shopping for groceries too. Just make sure you don't have high calorie, poor nutrition foods in your favourites list!

25: Grocery Lists

A grocery list is likely to help you eat more healthily.

A study by Monash University[45] (Australia) found that using detailed meal plans and a grocery list to make the meals could have a meaningful impact on weight loss and long-term health among overweight and obese individuals.

Notice here that the study is combining meal planning with a grocery list.

One study[46] on low-income individuals found:

"Shopping with a list may be a useful tool for low-income individuals to improve diet or decrease body mass index."

Of course, it's not enough to write your grocery list. You need to stick to it. Beware of special offers when you get to the supermarket. Special offers can look really tempting, but the reality is that often they don't actually save you that much money.

Psychologists have spent a lot of time helping supermarkets sell their most profitable goods, so most of these will be displayed at eye level. Look on the lower shelves for good value products.

26: Reusable Shopping Bags

Research[47] by Uma R. Karmarkar (Harvard University, USA) and Bryan Bollinger (Duke University, USA) showed:

"Grocery store shoppers who bring their own bags are more likely to purchase organic produce and other healthy food. But those same shoppers often feel virtuous, because they are acting in an environmentally responsible way. That feeling easily persuades them that, because they are being good to the environment, they should treat themselves to cookies or potato chips or some other product with lots of fat, salt, or sugar."

You should still take bags with you when you go shopping, just be aware that doing that doesn't justify that extra snack purchase.

I've included this rather bizarre research finding, because it highlights a recurring theme of research. You are "good" and so you "reward" yourself with the type of food that is going to make you feel far from good in the long run. Of course, an occasional treat is fine. Check out Hack 170 for other ways to reward yourself.

27: Food Shopping

Brian Wansink[48] a researcher on behaviour change says:

"Most of us know that it's a bad personal policy to go shopping on an empty stomach. We think it's because we buy more food when we're hungry—but we don't. In our studies of starving shoppers, they buy the exact same amount of food as stuffed shoppers. They don't buy more, but they buy worse.

"When we're hungry, we buy foods that are convenient enough to eat right away and stop our cravings. We don't go for broccoli and tilapia; we go for carbs in a box or bag. We go for one of the "Four Cs": crackers, chips, cereal, or candy. We want packages we can open and eat from with our right hand while we drive home with our left."

He goes on to say:

"My colleague Aner Tal and I discovered this when we gave gum to shoppers at the start of their shopping trip. When we reconnected with them at the end of their trip, they rated themselves as less hungry and less tempted by food--and in another study we found they also bought 7 percent less junk food then those who weren't chewing gum."

So, two hacks in one – don't shop when hungry and chew gum while you are grocery shopping.

And here's a third one[49] from this researcher:

"The Miracle of Duct-Tape: When it's used at home, you become MacGyver. When it's used to divide your grocery cart, you become healthier. People who shop with divided carts that suggest they put their fruits and vegetables in the front buy 23 percent more of them. Do it yourself. Divide your cart with your coat, your purse, or your briefcase. Or bring your own duct tape."

28: Using A Mobile Phone

A study published in the Journal of the Academy of Marketing Science[50] found that when shoppers used a mobile phone in store for conversations unrelated to shopping it often resulted in an increase in unplanned purchases.

Dr Michael Sciandra, corresponding author of the study said:

"Our finding that phone use that is unrelated to shopping negatively affects shopping behaviour was in stark contrast to beliefs held by consumers. The vast majority of shoppers we asked thought that mobile phones did not have any negative effect."

The research does not say what additional purchases people made, but it's not a stretch to think it wouldn't be broccoli!

So, put your phone away while you are food shopping, even if you're like most of the responders to this study and you think it has no effect at all.

29: Help With Binge Eating

B ach Flower Remedies have been around for a long time. They are gentle remedies made from flowers and are designed to work on your emotions.

A study using them was conducted at the Clinical Research Unit of the Medical School of São Paulo State University, Brazil. The results were published in the *Journal of Alternative and Complementary Medicine*[51].

The researchers wanted to see how effective flower therapy was for anxiety in overweight or obese adults. They carried out a randomised placebo-controlled clinical trial.

Half the participants were given a mixture of Bach Flower Remedies:

- Impatiens for tension and anxiety

- White Chestnut for repetitive thoughts

- Cherry Plum for impulsive or compulsive attitudes

- Chicory for control and possessiveness

- Crab Apple for inaccurate perceptions including of your own self-image

- Pine for feelings of guilt and regret

The other half were given a placebo.

The study lasted four weeks and the researchers found "an improvement in indices related to anxiety, sleep patterns, and binge eating" in the study group.

While this study concentrated on binge eating, Bach Flower Remedies are very much worth a try even if you don't binge.

There are other Bach Flower remedies that might be appropriate for you. For example, if you comfort eat to suppress emotions and stay cheerful, take the Bach Flower remedy Agrimony.

These simple, safe remedies based on flowers have been in use for over fifty years. They're safe to take, even if you're taking medication. You can get this and other Bach Flower remedies from health stores and online.

30: Candies & Cookies

Professor Brian Wansink[52] and colleagues conducted a study with Kisses, a type of candy. They were put into containers. Some containers were opaque, and some were clear. Some were on the person's desk and some containers were 6 feet (1.8 metres) away. You guessed what happened, didn't you?

Participants ate an average of 7.7 Kisses each day when the chocolates were in clear containers on their desks; 4.6 when in opaque containers on the desk; 5.6 when in clear jars six feet away; and 3.1 when in opaque jars six feet away.

What was surprising was that the women consistently thought they ate more when they had to get up to get them. This suggests, Wansink said, that you are likely to eat fewer cookies in the cupboard versus those on the counter for two reasons. They take more effort to get, and you tend to think you ate more than you did.

So now you know what to do, don't you? Don't keep your unhealthy snacks in your desk drawer. Instead put them in a cupboard. At home put snacks in places that are more difficult to access. Store all your snacks in opaque rather than clear containers.

31: Omega 3 Fatty Acids

Many dieters believe that restricting fats in their diet is a good thing to do. Check out Hack 101 for more on this.

Research on one type of oil (omega 3 fatty acids) is showing big potential benefits for those who want to lose weight.

Jonathan D. Buckleyand[53] and Peter R. C. Howe of the University of South Australia reviewed the research and found:

"... in human studies there is a growing body of evidence indicating that increasing the intake of LC n-3 PUFA by 0.3–3.0 g/day can reduce body weight and body fat in overweight and obese individuals."

They go on to say:

"... there is still much controversy because the majority of studies have been of relatively short duration and the magnitude of the improvements have been modest. Accordingly, there is an urgent need for longer-term studies to determine the relative effects of EPA and DHA supplementation on body composition and the feasibility of using LC n-3 PUFA supplementation as a strategy to improve body composition in overweight and obese populations."

Another study supported this view. This was by Shichun Du[54] and colleagues from the Department of Endocrinology, Shanghai Xin Hua Hospital affiliated to Shanghai Jiao Tong University School of Medicine, Shanghai, China found:

"... we cannot obtain effective proof that fish oil intakes may decrease body weight in overweight/obese adults. However, it may help reduce the waist hip ratio especially when combined with life modification interventions. Because of the limited follow-up duration, the results should be treated with caution. Further large-scale research over a long time is needed to determine definitive conclusions."

Omega 3 oils can be found in fish and other seafood (especially cold-water fatty fish, such as salmon, mackerel, tuna, herring, and sardines) and in nuts (especially walnuts) and seeds (such as flaxseed and chia seeds). There are also useful amounts in some oils such as soybean oil, and canola oil.

A double-blind, randomised, controlled trial[55] of overweight and obese participants with type 2 diabetes showed the benefits of chia seeds. Both the active group and the control group were on a calorie-restricted diet, but the active group took 30 gm of salba-chia [a trademarked form of chia seeds] per day and the control group a placebo. The researchers concluded:

"The results of this study, support the beneficial role of Salba-chia seeds in promoting weight loss and improvements of obesity related risk factors, while maintaining good glycemic control."

When people want to increase their intake of omega 3 through supplementation, they often look to fish oil supplements. Fish don't make omega 3 oils in their bodies. They eat algae which contain omega 3 oils. Some fish, of course, don't eat algae themselves, but consume other fish that eat algae.

There have been concerns about heavy metals, such as mercury, in fish and fish oil supplements. Buying supplements made from algae goes straight to the source of the omega 3, rather than fish oils which use the fish as the middleman. It also reduces the risk of contamination, as the algae are usually grown in special vats and are not harvested directly from the sea. It may also reduce the risk of the oil being rancid. Much fish oil comes from South America and the long distances increase the chance of the oil being rancid[56]. Oil from algae is often produced more locally.

I started taking an omega 3 algae supplement a couple of years ago. I buy the one from Nothing Fishy[57], because it's from algae. I bought it because of the general health benefits of omega 3 supplements and had not thought about it effecting my appetite. After a time, I noticed that I felt more in control of my diet, I but didn't attribute it to the omega 3 capsules. (At this point I didn't know about the research I've written about here.)

Over time I became less regular in taking them, and my control of my appetite seemed to lessen, but I didn't connect the two. I started taking them again and my appetite control came back. This happened a few times before I made the connection.

This is, of course, a personal anecdote and doesn't mean it will work like this for everyone. Most of the research has been done using fish oil supplements rather than algae supplements but check out Hack 32 on chocolate cravings.

Also be aware that more is not always better. Make sure you follow the manufacturer's recommendation if you take an omega 3 supplement.

32: Chocolate Craving

Many good intentions can disappear in the face of chocolate. If you struggle to resist chocolate, try this hack.

A study in the *International Archives of Addiction Research and Medicine* whether flaxseed oil supplements (1000 mg per day) could help. Flaxseed oil is rich in omega 3 oils.

Pedro Luis Prior[58] and colleagues from the Universidade Federal de São Paulo, Brazil conducted a double blind, placebo-controlled, randomised trial. This meant that neither the participants nor the researchers interacting with them knew whether they were getting flaxseed oil capsules or a placebo that looked like it.

The Binge Eating Scale (BES) was applied before supplementation and at the end of the study (two months) in order to determine if there was any change in chocolate consumption. After the treatment, there was a significant difference between the BES scores only in the omega 3 group before and after the intervention. The researchers concluded:

"... our results suggest that omega 3 fatty acids may be important in mitigating chocolate craving and consumption."

If that doesn't work for you try this. Many years ago I was told/read that a craving for chocolate could be offset by taking extra zinc either as a supplement or in food. Foods that are rich in zinc include sunflower seeds, pumpkin seeds, tahini and green leafy vegetables.

Over the years I've told various people about this hack, and most have told me that it works well. So, even though I can't find any scientific evidence to back it up, I'm including it here.

Omega 3 and zinc have many important functions in the body, so topping up with these if you are deficient will help not only with chocolate cravings, but also with other aspects of wellbeing.

33: Diet Soda

M any people drink diet sodas, believing that this is a good thing to do. It seems a no-brainer. You will be saving calories by drinking a diet drink rather than the regular version.

Research shows it may not be as simple as that. Professor Ruopeng An[59] of the University of Illinois (USA) examined the dietary habits of more than 22,000 U.S. adults. He found that diet-beverage consumers may compensate for the absence of calories in their drinks by eating extra food that is loaded with sugar, sodium, fat and cholesterol.

An said:

"It may be that people who consume diet beverages feel justified in eating more, so they reach for a muffin or a bag of chips ... Or perhaps, in order to feel satisfied, they feel compelled to eat more of these high-calorie foods."

Susan E. Swithers[60] of Purdue University, USA offers an alternative possibility. She argues that diet soda may interfere with the learned relationships between sweet tastes and feelings of fulness, because diet soda provides the sweetness without a later sense of fulness. This may mean that when foods/drinks sweetened with sucrose or glucose are eaten, the body does not register the fullness from them, and so the person consumes more. She says:

"... negative consequences of ASB [artificially sweetened beverages] should not be interpreted to suggest that sugars should be consumed in preference to artificial sweeteners. Instead, consumption of artificial sweeteners may exacerbate the negative effects of sugars by reducing the ability to predict the consequences of consuming sugars reliably and/or by altering cognitive processes that lead to overconsumption."

Diet soda has been associated with heart disease, kidney disease and depression. We cannot say that diet soda causes these problems. It could be that people with these problems are more likely to consume diet soda. Another possibility is that overweight people are more likely to drink diet soda and are more likely to suffer from these illnesses.

The definitive research isn't available, but in the meantime be wary of diet sodas even if you are trying to lose weight.

34: Artificial Sweeteners

I f you can't give up sugar, do you think you are doing the right thing replacing it with artificial sweeteners? You could be wrong.

Researchers from the University of Manitoba (Canada) published a study in the *Canadian Medical Association Journal*[61]. They conducted a systematic review of 37 studies that followed over 400,000 people for an average of 10 years. Only seven of these studies were randomized controlled trials (the gold standard in clinical research), involving 1003 people followed for 6 months on average.

The trials did not show a consistent effect of artificial sweeteners on weight loss. In fact, almost the opposite. The longer observational studies showed a link between consumption of artificial sweeteners and relatively higher risks of weight gain and obesity, high blood pressure, diabetes, heart disease and other health issues.

Researcher Dr. Ryan Zarychanski, Assistant Professor, Rady Faculty of Health Sciences, University of Manitoba said:

"We found that data from clinical trials do not clearly support the intended benefits of artificial sweeteners for weight management."

Another study[62] suggested that artificial sweeteners may alter the gut biome in a way that can lead to dysbiosis, with fewer healthy gut bacteria. (See Hack 62 Gut Biome to understand how important this is.)

Belinda Lennerz[63] (Boston Children's Hospital, USA) and Jochen K. Lennerz (Massachusetts General Hospital, USA) write in the academic journal *Clinical Chemistry*:

"... artificial sweeteners have been shown to alter food reward and food cravings in some but not all studies."

The evidence for artificial sweeteners being beneficial for weight loss is far from clear. There is increasing evidence that they may be detrimental.

Try to wean yourself off sugar rather than switching to sweeteners or sugar-free drinks. If you're already using artificial sweeteners and diet drinks work to reduce or eliminate them.

35: It's My Job!

Some people believe they are overweight because of the amount they need to eat out because of work or other commitments.

At first sight this is a reasonable thing to say but think about famous people who eat out a lot – heads of state, royalty and celebrities. Are they all overweight? They've found a way to do it. You can too.

Eating out a lot may make it more difficult to control your weight, but it's not impossible.

If possible, check out a restaurant menu before you go. See what foods will work for you. Consider whether you want to ask the staff if a dish can be modified in some way. Don't forget when you get there to start with a big glass of water. See Hack 58.

36: What Are Your Triggers?

The US Centers For Disease Control[64] has some great advice:

"Create a list of "cues" by reviewing your food diary [see Hack 72] to become more aware of when and where you're "triggered" to eat for reasons other than hunger. Note how you are typically feeling at those times. Often an environmental "cue", or a particular emotional state, is what encourages eating for non-hunger reasons. Common triggers for eating when not hungry are:

- Opening up the cabinet and seeing your favorite snack food.

- Sitting at home watching television.

- Before or after a stressful meeting or situation at work.

- Coming home after work and having no idea what's for dinner.

- Having someone offer you a dish they made "just for you!" [See hack 147]

- Walking past a candy dish on the counter.

- Sitting in the break room beside the vending machine.

- Seeing a plate of doughnuts at the morning staff meeting.

- Swinging through your favorite drive-through every morning.

- Feeling bored or tired and thinking food might offer a pick-me-up.

"Circle the "cues" on your list that you face on a daily or weekly basis. While the Thanksgiving holiday may be a trigger to overeat, for now focus on cues you face more often. Eventually you want a plan for as many eating cues as you can.

"Ask yourself these questions for each "cue" you've circled:

"Is there anything I can do to avoid the cue or situation?

"This option works best for cues that don't involve others. For example, could you choose a different route to work to avoid stopping at a fast food restaurant on the way? Is there another place in the break room where you can sit so you're not next to the vending machine?

"For things I can't avoid, can I do something differently that would be healthier?

"Obviously, you can't avoid all situations that trigger your unhealthy eating habits, like staff meetings at work. In these situations, evaluate your options. Could you suggest or bring healthier snacks or beverages? Could you offer to take notes to distract your attention? Could you sit farther away from the food so it won't be as easy to grab something? Could you plan ahead and eat a healthy snack before the meeting?"

Great advice from the CDC.

The website www.healthcareevolve.ca[65] also offers ideas on replacing your triggers.

"… identifying your cue will be key, then brainstorming how you can alter it will come next. It might be as simple as walking through a different door to your house when you come home, or instead of walking inside immediately after parking your car, you throw on your runners and go for a walk."

Robert Taibbi[66] writing in *Psychology Today* has these suggestions:

"… when you realize, while driving home, that you are stressed, … you deliberately sit in the car and listen to music that you like while sitting in the driveway, or do a few minutes of deep breathing to relax, rather than automatically marching into the danger-zone of the kitchen."

Tackle one cue at a time, otherwise you are likely to feel overwhelmed.

37:
Carbohydrate-Insulin Model

Many authorities argue that weight loss is simple: eat fewer calories than you use, and you'll lose weight. They may recognise that people many find it hard to do, but it's still fairly straight-forward.

But there are alternative views which are gaining ground.

Dr. David Ludwig[67], Professor at Harvard Medical School (USA) and colleagues have proposed an alternative process. They have published a paper "The Carbohydrate-Insulin Model: A Physiological Perspective on the Obesity Pandemic" in The *American Journal of Clinical Nutrition*.

Rather than urge people to eat less, a strategy which usually doesn't work in the long run, the carbohydrate-insulin model suggests another path that focuses more on what we eat.

The carbohydrate-insulin model suggests that the current obesity epidemic is due, in part, to hormonal responses to changes in food quality. Foods with a high glycaemic index fundamentally change metabolism.

The glycaemic index ranks carbohydrates on a scale from 0 to 100 based on how quickly and how much they raise blood sugar levels after eating. Foods with a high glycemic index, like white bread, are rapidly digested and cause substantial fluctuations in blood sugar. Foods with a low glycemic index, like whole oats, are digested more slowly, prompting a more gradual rise in blood sugar.

High glycaemic foods include:

- sugar and sugary foods

- sugary soft drinks

- white bread

- potatoes

- white rice

- Refined breakfast cereal

- Sugar-sweetened beverages

- Couscous

- White-flour pasta

Low glycaemic foods include:
- Apple

- Orange

- Kidney beans

- Black beans

- Lentils

- Wheat tortilla

- Cashews

- Peanuts

- Carrots

Eating low glycaemic foods can help reduce cravings and reduce mood swings and headaches. Make sure you add these to your diet.

There are books and websites that have comprehensive lists of foods and their glycaemic index.

The University of Sydney (Australia) maintains a searchable database[68] of foods and their corresponding glycaemic indices.

High glycaemic foods demand a greater insulin response. This may increase body fat and weight and lead to insulin resistance and to exhaustion of endocrine pancreatic function.

The authors believe that focusing on what you eat rather than how much you eat is a better strategy for weight management.

Harvard School of Public Health[69] says:

"Eating many high-glycaemic-index foods – which cause powerful spikes in blood sugar – can lead to an increased risk for type 2 diabetes and heart disease. There is also preliminary work linking high-glycaemic diets to age-related macular degeneration, ovulatory infertility and colorectal cancer."

A study[70] in *The American Journal of Clinical Nutrition* looked at overweight and obsess young men and found that:

"a high-GI meal decreased plasma glucose, increased hunger, and selectively stimulated brain regions associated with reward and craving in the late postprandial period"

The postprandial period is the four hours after the meal. This suggests that eating a high glycaemic meal can mean you are likely to experience greater hunger than if you consume a low-glycaemic meal of similar calories, macronutrient and palatability.

Although there are researchers who dispute the carbohydrate-insulin model of weight management, the wider benefits of eating a diet with very few high glycaemic foods suggests that you should be moving to this type of diet anyway.

38: Write Yourself A Letter

W rite yourself a letter and give it to a trusted friend to post it back to you in 3 or 6 months. They don't need to read the letter – give it to them sealed.

In the letter write about what you want to achieve in the next 3/6 months. Think about how you want to feel and what you want to have done, as well as what you want to weigh. List the new habits you want to be embedded in your life by then.

You can also use the website www.futureme.org[71] – here you write an email to yourself to be sent to you in one year or longer. The system then automatically sends it to you on the correct date. Don't change your email in the meantime!

The knowledge that you will be receiving a letter/email from your past self can help you persevere when motivation is low.

39: Make A Commitment To Yourself

The US Centers For Disease Control[72] says:

"Making the decision to lose weight, change your lifestyle, and become healthier is a big step. Start by making a commitment to yourself. Many people find it helpful to sign a written contract committing to the process. This contract may include how much weight you want to lose, the date you'd like to lose the weight by, changes you'll make to establish healthy eating patterns, and a plan for regular physical activity.

"Writing down the reasons you want to lose weight can also help. It might be because you have a family history of heart disease, or because you want to see your kids get married, or because you want to feel better in your clothes. Post these reasons where they serve as a daily reminder of why you want to make this change."

You could write this on a computer or on paper. It has been suggested that writing on paper has more impact, so consider whether this is likely to be true for you.

40: Self-Respect

T his hack goes by the name of "self interventions". Self affirmations aren't the same as the affirmations in Hack 42.

Claude Steele originally popularised self-affirmation theory in the late 1980s. It remains a well-studied theory in social psychological research. Self-affirmation theory says that if individuals reflect on values that are personally relevant to them, they are less likely to experience distress and react defensively when confronted with information that contradicts or threatens their sense of self.

How is this of use if you want to lose weight? It's well-known that when people are faced with information designed to change their behaviour, they often respond defensively. They find ways of ignoring or justifying their existing attitudes and behaviour. Faced with the information that you should eat fewer fast-food meals, do you dig in and ignore it or find a reason to dismiss the message as untrue?

In self-affirmation interventions people are encouraged to write about their values. Researchers[73] have found that this reduces defensive responses and encourages change.

There are lots of lists of values that you can use. Just search the internet for "list of values".

Here are some that might be relevant to weight loss:

- Acceptance

- Balance

- Comfort

- Curiosity

- Determination

- Forgiveness

- Generosity

- Honesty

- Independence

- Patience

- Respect

- Gratitude

Pick one of these values and spend some time writing about it, and its relationship to your desire to weigh less. On another day read what you've written. You may want to add to it. You may want to choose another value.

Addressing your values in this way can make you more open to change and more motivated to change.

You can also think about values rather than goals. www.healthcareevolve.ca[74] suggests:

"Instead of saying, 'I want to lose 20 pounds.' How about, 'I want to be healthier or lose weight, so I can keep up with my kids, so I can have less pain in my knees, so I can enjoy my retirement, so I can live the life I want to live…'"

41: Stress

Research psychologist Sarah Jackson[75] (University College London, UK) says:

"People tend to report overeating and "comfort eating" foods that are high in sugar, fat and calories when stressed. And because the stress hormone cortisol plays a role in metabolism and fat storage, there are plausible biological mechanisms behind a possible link between stress and putting on weight.

"In research published in *Obesity* we found that chronic stress was consistently linked with people being more heavily, and more persistently, overweight."

This study measured cortisol levels in the hair as a better measure of chronic stress than blood levels would be.

What happens to you when you're stressed? A few people eat less, but most people eat more. If you're one of those people who eat more, a useful approach might be to find ways of making your life less stressful or handling the stress you do have better.

At this point you may be thinking "easier said than done!"

You have to be pro-active to reduce the stress in your life or handle it better. There isn't just one strategy that works for everyone.

The UK NHS website[76] says:

"The most unhelpful thing you can do is turn to something unhealthy to help you cope, such as smoking or drinking."

If you're feeling overwhelmed with too much to do, check out Hack 182.

Find a therapist to help you, if you feel that you don't have enough support – see Hacks 122 to 129 or join a support group (Hack 130).

Exercise has been proven over and over to be a good stress buster. Check out Hack 45 if you hate the thought of exercise.

Volunteering can reduce your blood pressure, make you grateful for the good things you have in your life, improve your self-worth, and even prolong your life. So that's another and different strategy to try.

Mindfulness (see Hack 53) has been shown to help with stress. Deep breathing and yoga (see Hack 129) can also help.

These are just some of the many strategies you can use to help counteract stress.

If you're struggling to lose weight, it may be time to put that on one side and concentrate on a more rounded view of what's going on in your life and what you can do about it.

42: New Way With Affirmations

Affirmations can be extremely useful in lots of situations. Affirmations are positive and stated in the present tense, as though they are true now. For example, "I choose and enjoy healthy food" would be a great affirmation. "I want to choose and enjoy healthy food" would be a poor one.

Once you have decided on your affirmation, you say it (or them) out loud several times a day. You may want to write them down and post them on your fridge and mirror too.

Caroline Rushforth, an NLP coach has written about how she found affirmations helpful in her plan to lose weight (www.mindbodygreen.com[77]):

"Going from negative self talk to self love doesn't happen overnight. However, using these affirmations over time, I noticed my thinking changed. And that's the first step."

In the article she lists 15 affirmations she used, such as:

- "I bring the qualities of fulfillment, happiness and contentment into my life as I am now.

- "I let go of any guilt I hold around food choices.

- "I accept my body for the shape I have been blessed with."

As well as using affirmations in this general way, you can also use them to address a tendency to snack frequently.

When you have finished your meal, say an affirmation out loud several times. Here are some suggestions:

- "I've now finished eating till lunch/dinner/6.00 pm." (whatever is suitable given the circumstances)

- "I have eaten enough food to last me till ..."

- "I'm full and do not need to eat till ..."

If you don't like these, vary it till you find one that is useful.

Positive affirmations are often uncomfortable to say to begin with but persevere and they will get easier and feel more natural.

43: Your Values

This hack goes by the name of "self interventions". Self affirmations aren't the same as the affirmations in Hack 42.

Claude Steele originally popularised self-affirmation theory in the late 1980s. It remains a well-studied theory in social psychological research. Self-affirmation theory says that if individuals reflect on values that are personally relevant to them, they are less likely to experience distress and react defensively when confronted with information that contradicts or threatens their sense of self.

How is this of use if you want to lose weight? It's well-known that when people are faced with information designed to change their behaviour, they often respond defensively. They find ways of ignoring or justifying their existing attitudes and behaviour. Faced with the information that you should eat fewer fast-food meals, do you dig in and ignore it or find a reason to dismiss the message as untrue?

In self-affirmation interventions people are encouraged to write about their values. Researchers[78] have found that this reduces defensive responses and encourages change.

There are lots of lists of values that you can use. Just search the internet for "list of values".

Here are some that might be relevant to weight loss:

- Acceptance

- Balance

- Comfort

- Curiosity

- Determination

- Forgiveness

- Generosity

- Honesty

- Independence

- Patience

- Respect

- Gratitude

Pick one of these values and spend some time writing about it, and its relationship to your desire to weigh less. On another day read what you've written. You may want to add to it. You may want to choose another value.

Addressing your values in this way can make you more open to change and more motivated to change.

You can also think about values rather than goals. www.healthcareevolve.ca[79] suggests:

"Instead of saying, 'I want to lose 20 pounds.' How about, 'I want to be healthier or lose weight, so I can keep up with my kids, so I can have less pain in my knees, so I can enjoy my retirement, so I can live the life I want to live…'"

44: Can You Lose Weight By Exercising?

"Exercise is a celebration of what your body can do. Not a punishment for what you ate."

Unfortunately, I don't know who first said this, but I know it hits the nail on the head of what our attitude to exercise should be.

Many people see exercise as a way of losing weight. That's their focus. They want to know:

- Does exercise help you lose weight faster?

- How many calories will this exercise consume?

- What type of exercise is best for losing weight?

- Is working out 30 minutes a day enough to lose weight?

- How much exercise to do I need to do because I've eaten a doughnut/ a tub of ice cream/ a bar of chocolate?

- If I go for a bike ride, can I stop and have a cake and coffee in the middle?

The questions are endless, but they all focus on the idea that exercise is about losing weight.

Learning to balance healthy eating and physical activity can help you lose weight more easily and keep it off.

The American Heart Association[80] says:

"Take it from people who have successfully maintained weight loss: "98% have modified their eating habits and 94% have increased their physical activity, especially walking."

Drs Caroline M. Apovian and Judith Korner write in the Journal of Clinical Endocrinology & Metabolism[81]:

"... exercise alone (without limiting calories) usually isn't enough to cause weight loss. But exercise plays an important part in helping people who have [lost] weight keep that weight off."

In other words, exercise should be part of your plan.

But are you deceiving yourself? The UK NHS says that 8 out of 10 people think they exercise enough, but in reality, only 3 out of 10 actually do. You should be doing at least 30 minutes five times a week.

Remember that there are many other reasons to exercise. Regular exercise is good for you. It helps to prevent chronic diseases. It's good for your mood and for your brain too. There are so many reasons to exercise regularly even if you don't want to lose weight.

Check out Hack 70 about the important role exercise plays in maintaining weight loss.

45: Hate Exercise

The last hack suggested that taking exercise can be part of an overall weight loss package. It seems to be particularly helpful for weight management.

Do you hate the thought of exercise? Lots of people do.

It may be that you were laughed at when you were at school because you weren't very sporty. Or maybe you were sporty, and you've put on a lot of weight and feel breathless and unfit now.

If you haven't exercised much, you may want to argue that exercise shows how weak, unhealthy and unfit you are. That is almost certainly true, yet that is an advantage. When you start exercising, you will rapidly improve if you're starting from a very low point. You will find you are making progress. That can be very motivating.

Rejoice in that. Don't just leap on the scales and judge your workout on how much weight you're losing. (In fact, to begin with, you may put on weight, as muscle weighs more than fat.)

Focus on how much faster or further you can run than you did last week or last month. Give yourself a pat on the back for the heavier weights you are lifting at the gym. Celebrate day by day that you are becoming more flexible.

Appreciate how you don't get out of breath at all/so much when you walk up the stairs. Notice how easy it is to lift your shopping out of the car or pick up your child. Feel pleased that you are less likely to fall. If you stumble, notice how much faster you can right yourself.

You may be thinking that you still hate exercise. You know it will be good for you, but you still don't want to do it.

Are you good at snacking? Lots of overweight people are. How about trying exercise snacking? These are small bursts of activity throughout the day. Try:

- Air squats while you're waiting for the kettle to boil.

- Standing on one leg while cleaning your teeth.

- Run up and down the stairs a few times.

- Do star jumps before and after washing dishes.

Get the idea?

Hopefully, you're thinking you could cope with exercise snacking. But maybe you're thinking: "Great idea, but I know I won't do it."

I was talking to a friend in her sixties, who told me she hates exercise. She knows she should do it but hates it. She said it almost as though that settled the matter. She didn't need to take any because she hated it.

Now that approach may be OK for not reading Tolstoy or not eating bananas, but it's really not OK when it comes to exercise.

But what would she have said to me if I'd said: "I hate cleaning my teeth, so I don't do it."

I think she would have been shocked. She would have thought that it didn't matter if I hated it, I still absolutely needed to clean my teeth to avoid bad breath and to prevent dental caries. She might have even told me that.

And, of course, she would have been right.

So, you could treat exercise as a necessary evil. It is something you need to do to keep your body and mind toned and strong.

I find the best way of dealing with unpleasant things that I need to do is to work out how much the time is as a proportion of my life.

For example, I'm going to assume for this calculation that I will live to be 90.

90 years = 47,304,000 Minutes

You can see what a small part of my life the current 30-minute workout would be (I'm not going to give you some impossible fraction here!)

You may want to experiment to find the type of exercise you hate the least! But just accept that you will always hate it, but that you will do it. You will focus on the results you will achieve rather than the time you spend doing the exercise.

46: Time For HIIPA

Emmanuel Stamatakis[82], Professor of Physical Activity, Lifestyle and Population Health (University of Sydney, Australia) published a paper in the *British Journal of Sports Medicine*. Stamatakis and colleagues argue that many daily tasks can be classified as 'high intensity' physical activity for less fit people. These are activities that get you out of breath enough to boost your fitness.

He calls these activities "high intensity incidental physical activity" (HIIPA). Activities may include washing the car, climbing stairs, carrying groceries, riding home from work and walking uphill. Whether or not an activity can be classified as HIIPA for you depends on how fit you are.

Professor Stamatakis says:

"There is a lot of research telling us that any type of HIIT [high intensity interval training], irrespective of the duration and number of repetitions is one of the most effective ways to rapidly improve fitness and cardiovascular health and HIIPA works on the same idea."

He proposes that significant health benefits could be gained by doing three to five brief HIIPA sessions totalling as little as five to 10 minutes a day, most days of the week.

Do you avoid strenuous daily activities? Do you get someone else to do them or use a machine? Maybe it's time to see the benefit of adding these to your daily life and doing them yourself.

47: Muscle Mass

Many people think about the calories they burn during exercise, but you can also burn extra calories at other times if you do resistance exercises, such as gym workouts.

If you have built more muscle through resistance training, your resting metabolic rate will be higher.

David R Clark[83] and colleagues from Liverpool John Moores University (UK) write:

"... muscle size plays a major role in determining resting metabolic rate (RMR), which is how many calories your body requires to function at rest. Resting metabolic rate accounts for 60-75% of total energy expenditure in non-exercising people, and fat is the body's preferred energy source at rest.

"Increasing muscle size through resistance training increases RMR, thereby increasing or sustaining fat loss over time. A review of 18 studies found that resistance training was effective at increasing resting metabolic rate, whereas aerobic exercise and combined aerobic and resistance exercise were not as effective."

In addition, you will use more calories immediately after exercise, as the body seeks to restore the muscles to their resting state.

Of course, if you use resistance training or other exercises as an excuse to eat a lot more, you are likely to put on weight, even though your resting metabolic rate is higher.

If you're a woman and now envisaging that you will have to become unattractively muscly to get the benefit, this is not true. Having good muscle mass will give you good muscle tone and enhance your muscle tone.

48: Putting On Weight As You Get Older?

Metabolism does slow, but not by the huge amount that many people think. Researchers[84] from Pennington Biomedical Research Center (USA) studied how metabolism changes with age. Four of these researchers were part of an international team of scientists who analysed the average calories burned by more than 6,600 people as they went about their daily lives. The participants' ages ranged from one week old to 95 years, and they lived in 29 different countries.

They found that our metabolisms don't really start to decline again until after age 60. The slowdown is gradual, only 0.7 percent a year. But it does mount up – eventually. A person in their 90s needs 26% fewer calories each day than someone in midlife.

Lost muscle mass as we get older may be partly to blame, the researchers say, since muscle burns more calories than fat. But it's not the whole picture.

One of the researchers, Dr Ravussin says:

"We took dwindling muscle mass into account. After 60, a person's cells slow down … This study shows that the work cells do changes over the course of the lifespan in ways we couldn't fully appreciate before."

So yes, your metabolism does slow down, but it's a small amount each year and is no excuse for piling on the pounds. There are other factors involved.

As we get older, we tend to exercise less. We may stop active sport. We just generally tend to move around less. Many people believe that it's natural to slow down and take it easy as we get older. But the opposite is true. Staying active helps us stay healthy.

As people get older, they often eat more from habit than from hunger. They eat a particular meal at a particular time because that's what they've always done and regardless of their appetite.

People who are at home all day often eat because of boredom or simply that the food is there. Try to change things around. Keep some healthy snacks easily available.

The Harvard Medical School[85] newsletter (USA) says that as we get older:

"We lose muscle mass and bone density, so while we may weigh the same as we used to, or even less (and congratulate ourselves on being thin), we may actually be lugging around more fat tissue. So we need to keep an eye on our waist size, not just our weight, especially after about age 50. Waist size is a fairly accurate reflection of how much visceral fat we've accumulated in our abdomens. And visceral fat is the metabolically active form of fat that causes so much harm."

The big change is the mental shift. Knowing that you don't have to get fatter as you get older. You know that your metabolism slows a bit, but that doesn't mean you have to put on a lot of weight.

49: I'll Start Monday

M any people start a diet on a Monday, but why?

The best reason is that you need to do some planning and preparation. You will have the time for that over the weekend. We know planning and preparation is essential for success, so good on you.

But do you say "I'll start Monday" for another reason?

Are you putting off the start date, maybe dreading it? If so, it probably means you're not ready to start. You need to work towards getting ready to start, not plan a date to start.

When you say: "I'll start Monday", does that mean you eat more between now and then? If so, you're probably not ready to start.

If you're in this position, consider doing one of the simple hacks and keeping your eating and exercising as it currently is. For example, try Hack 92 A Simple Way to Reduce Cravings or Hack 85 Choose A Plate With A Wide Rim.

50: Stop Clock Watching!

D o you often eat from habit? Do you eat according to the clock? When asked; "Are you hungry?", do you immediately look at the time to decide the answer?

Because it's 11 am, do you decide that you'll have a milky coffee and a couple of biscuits? That's just what happens at 11am.

Perhaps we shouldn't call it a decision, as it's so automatic.

So, when someone asks: "are you hungry?", don't look at your watch, but check out how you feel. When you notice it's your normal lunchtime, stop and think what you want to eat according to how hungry you are. This will take practice and perseverance.

Be aware that for some people this hack doesn't work. Years of dieting have messed up their sense of when they are hungry. Try checking in with yourself to see if you are hungry but be prepared to abandon this strategy if you always get "yes" regardless of the time of day.

51: Do You Eat Out Of Habit?

D o you always have a similar size meal for lunch regardless of what you ate in the morning?

Do you always have a pudding or other dessert with your dinner?

Do you always have bread with soup?

Do you always have a bar of chocolate or a couple of glasses of wine in the evening?

Do you do some of your eating out of habit? Look for your food habits and experiment by changing them.

52: Make New Habits – Any Habits

When you think about changing habits in relation to losing weight, you probably think about habits related to weight management – no food after a certain time in the evening, one biscuit instead of two with your morning coffee, etc.

But an interesting study by Gina Cleo[86] of Bond University (Australia) showed that changing <u>any</u> small habits can help your weight. Her research published in the *International Journal of Obesity* recruited 75 participants with excess weight or obesity and randomised them into three groups.

One program promoted breaking old habits, one promoted forming new habits, and one group was a control (no intervention). She explained:

"The habit-breaking group was sent a text message with a different task to perform every day. These tasks were focused on breaking usual routines and included things such as "drive a different way to work today", "listen to a new genre of music" or "write a short story".

"The habit-forming group was asked to follow a program that focused on forming habits centred around healthy lifestyle changes. The group was encouraged to incorporate ten healthy tips into their daily routine, so they became second-nature."

You may be surprised at the results:

"After 12 weeks, the habit-forming and habit-breaking participants had lost an average of 3.1kg. More importantly, after 12 months of no intervention and no contact, they had lost another 2.1kg on average."

The author does not explain why the habit-breaking worked even though it was not related to weight loss. It may well be that changing habits gave the participants a sense that they were more in control of their life and so they made more healthful decisions.

See also Hack 183 Create A Ritual for more of this type of approach.

53: Mindful Eating

M indfulness is a practice based on Zen Buddhism. It has become popular as a way of self-calming. The practice focuses on purposely bringing your attention into the present moment without judgement.

Many people find a mindfulness approach helps to change their thoughts and behaviours around food.

It's not about forcing yourself to behave in a certain way or setting restrictions on what you do. It's about learning to understand and recognise your relationship with food at any time without judging or criticising yourself.

This is difficult for many people and needs effort to achieve it. There are many apps and courses to help. Personally, I like the Headspace app[87].

A research study[88] by Hugo J.E.M. Alberts (Maastricht University, Netherlands) and colleagues offers support for the effectiveness of mindfulness training. The study examined whether mindfulness-based strategies can effectively reduce food cravings in an overweight and obese adult population.

Individuals participating in a dietary group treatment for overweight received an additional 7-week manual-based training that aimed to promote regulation of cravings by means of acceptance. The control group did not receive this additional training program.

The results showed that participants in the experimental group reported significantly lower cravings for food after the intervention compared to the control group.

Another project[89] which reviewed many studies on mindfulness and eating involving college students concluded:

"higher levels of mindfulness have been found to be associated with lower emotional eating and binge eating in students than in their less mindful peers."

McGill University[90] (Canada) researchers surveyed existing research in this area and concluded:

"Interventions based on mindfulness proved "moderately effective for weight loss" and "largely effective in reducing obesity-related eating behaviours.""

They also found that interventions based on mindfulness led to less weight loss during the active phase of studies, but that participants continued to lose weight after the active phase. This is often the time when people who have lost weight through dieting start to put it on again.

The Association of UK Dietitians[91] (BDA) offer some support for mindful eating, but also a warning too:

"Eating mindfully is a way to enjoy what you're eating whilst being attuned with your body and acknowledging your thoughts and feelings. It can help encourage positive eating behaviours and healthy eating choices as you choose foods that are nourishing as well as satisfying to your body.

"This approach may not be suitable for those with an active eating disorder. Mindful eating can lead to justification of undereating and can be harmful to those recovering from eating disorders and disordered eating. Mindful eating is of limited use to people with Anorexia, because of their need for distraction from, rather than increased awareness of eating behaviours."

If this doesn't apply to you, then you may find trying mindfulness training really helpful.

54: Mindfully Eating A Raisin

UC Berkeley's Greater Good Science Center (USA), in collaboration with HopeLab, launched the website Greater Good in Action. It has lots of resources. Here's how the website[92] describes the raisin eating exercise:

"One of the most basic and widely used methods for cultivating mindfulness is to focus your attention on each of your senses as you eat a raisin. This simple exercise is often used as an introduction to the practice of mindfulness. In addition to increasing mindfulness more generally, the raisin meditation can promote mindful eating and foster a healthier relationship with food. Try it with a single raisin—you might find that it's the most delicious raisin you've ever eaten."

Professor Jon Kabat-Zinn offers a detailed script for this – you can find it on his website mbsrtraining.com[93]. He has it as an audio tract and as a written script. The script starts:

"Place a few raisins in your hand. If you don't have raisins, any food will do. Imagine that you have just come to Earth from a distant planet without such food. Now, with this food in hand, you can begin to explore it with all of your senses."

This short exercise encourages you to be present with what you are eating. It shows you how you can learn to eat more mindfully – not just raisins but everything else. You may be surprised at just how satisfied you feel after eating a raisin in this way.

55: Intuitive Eating

Intuitive Eating (IE) was created in 1995 by two registered dietitians, Evelyn Tribole and Elyse Resch, based on their extensive experience working with clients.

Evelyn Tribole[94] says:

"Intuitive Eating is an evidenced-based, mind-body health approach, comprised of 10 Principles ... It is a weight-neutral model with a validated assessment scale and over 90 studies to date ... "

Intuitive Eating is not just eating when you are hungry and stopping when you are full. There are ten principles of intuitive eating:

- Principle 1: Reject the Diet Mentality

- Principle 2: Honor Your Hunger

- Principle 3: Make Peace with Food

- Principle 4: Challenge the Food Police

- Principle 5: Discover the Satisfaction Factor

- Principle 6: Feel Your Fullness

- Principle 7: Cope with Your Emotions with Kindness

- Principle 8: Respect Your Body

- Principle 9: Movement—Feel the Difference

- Principle 10: Honor Your Health with Gentle Nutrition

Like the idea of this approach? You can find out more on the website intuitiveeatin g.org[95]. They have a list of counsellors trained in their method on the website too. Also look out for books by Evelyn Tribole and Elyse Resch.

An article by Muriel Nogué and colleagues in the *American Journal of Clinical Nutrition*[96] confirmed that this was a useful approach for women who had undergone bariatric surgery:

"This study highlights a significant association between intuitive eating and BMI [body mass index] decrease after bariatric surgery."

56: The Mindless Margin

Often weight gain happens slowly over the years. You gradually put on weight for no obvious reason.

Behavioural researcher Brian Wansink[97] says:

"If we eat way too little, we know it. If we eat way too much, we know it. But there is a calorie range – a Mindless Margin– where we feel fine and are unaware of small differences. That is, the difference between 1900 calories and 2000 calories is one we cannot detect, nor can we detect the difference between 2000 and 2100 calories. But over the course of a year, this mindless margin would either cause us to lose ten pounds or to gain ten pounds. It takes 3500 extra calories to equal one pound. It does not matter if we eat these extra 3500 calories in one week or gradually over the entire year. They will all add up to one pound."

He goes on to say:

"This is the silver lining to this dark, cloudy sky. The same things that lead us to mindlessly gain weight can also help us mindlessly lose weight."

So, eating 100 calories a day less will mean that you will gradually lose weight. It won't be spectacular, but it could be consistent and relatively easy to do.

Of course, many diet gurus offer amazing transformations in as little as 12 weeks. That may be a more attractive option, but you are likely to put the weight on again afterwards.

The Mayo Clinic[98] says:

"The concern with fast weight loss is that it usually takes extraordinary efforts in diet and exercise — efforts that could be unhealthy and that you probably can't maintain as permanent lifestyle changes."

Also, check out Hack 185 Radical Change. This looks at how reasonable it is to think you can make massive changes quickly.

57: When Others Are Unhelpful

R elationships can be difficult when you are wanting to change. Hopefully the people around you want to support you and help you to lose and manage your weight.

But sometimes this doesn't happen. There can be various reasons for that. Sadly, it can end up with big arguments or you give in because that's the easiest thing to do.

It can be difficult to say no to tasty high calorie treats when someone keeps offering them to you. It's hard to limit your alcohol intake if the other person keeps topping up your glass.

The situation can become a real battleground, which doesn't help. We know being stressed leads to a lot of people eating more.

Instead of shouting and fighting, use three simple words:

"Please humour me."

Say them in a calm voice, or as calm a voice as you can manage.

This takes the heat out of the situation. You're not asking the other person to back down or admit they are being selfish or feeling scared.

You're just asking them to go along with you and what you want. It won't work every time, but it will work sometimes.

58: Water Before Meals

E lizabeth A Dennis[99] and colleagues conducted an experiment in which half the participants drank 500 ml (1.06 US pints) of water before meals. After 12 weeks weight loss was around 2 kg (4.4 lb) greater in the water group than in the non-water group. This was a 44% greater decline in weight over the 12 weeks for participants who drank water before meals.

All the participants were middle-aged and older adults and followed a low-calorie diet for the 12 weeks. There is every reason to think this would apply whatever your age and whether or not you are reducing your calories.

Another study by Helen M. Parretti[100] (University of Birmingham, UK) and colleagues came to a similar conclusion. The results were published in the academic journal *Obesity*. Obese participants, who were instructed to consume 500 ml of water 30 min before main meals, lost 1.3 kg more than the control group in the 12 weeks that the study was carried out. Neither group knew that the research was about water or what the other group was doing.

Dr Alex Ruani[101] of University College London (UK) is also an advocate of drinking water before a meal. She says that drinking water prior to meals will help keep the stomach feeling fuller for longer.

This is a really cheap and easy hack, so do try it.

59: Water And Metabolism

The previous hack shows how beneficial it is to drink water before your meals. But there's mounting evidence that drinking more water generally is beneficial.

John Hopkins University[102] (USA) says:

"After all, 60% of your body is composed of water, meaning that the clear, calorie-free liquid plays a role in just about every bodily function. The more hydrated you are, research suggests, the more efficiently your body works at tasks that range from thinking to burning body fat."

The website Physicians Weight Loss Centers[103] says:

"Water is involved with almost every biological function in the body, so therefore your body's metabolism slows down in a dehydrated state. When your body does not have adequate amounts of water, your calorie burning machines (muscles) slow down dramatically. Over 70% of your muscle consists of water, so when they are not fully hydrated their ability to generate energy is severely inhibited.

"Another important factor to understand is – your body's ability to utilize fat as fuel is also restricted when you are in a dehydrated state."

A study of overweight volunteers in the *Journal Of Clinical And Diagnostic Research*[104] concluded:

"The decrease in body weight, body mass index and body composition scores of overweight subjects at the end of study period establishes the role of water induced thermogenesis in weight reduction of overweight subjects."

Before you get excited and think drinking more water is your new weight control plan, the number of calories involved is very small. It will not be enough on its own. Of course, there are all sorts of other health reasons to drink plenty of water, so this is a thing you should do regardless.

The Heart Research Institute UK[105] gives another reason to drink more water:

"If you really need to have some hand-to-mouth action, then carry a water bottle with you and sip on it regularly. It can really help satisfy the need to snack on food. It will also ensure you stay well hydrated, which can help keep you better in control of your appetite. Dehydration will make you hungrier and thirsty and more likely to eat or drink something high in energy even if you don't need it."

60: Yo-Yo Dieting

Yo-yo dieting, also called weight cycling and episodic weight loss, is a pattern of losing weight and then regaining it.

It is commonly thought that yo-yo dieting leads ultimately to weight gain and a "messed up metabolism".

The scientific evidence for this is far from conclusive, although some researchers are convinced it is the case.

Tim Spector[106], Professor of Genetic Epidemiology, King's College London (UK) explains:

"People who regularly go on diets tend to lose weight initially but bounce back and even gain weight after stopping the regime. This phenomenon – dubbed yo-yo dieting – is associated with changes in metabolism and is one reason why the vast majority of calorie-based diets fail... Previous studies in identical twins who differed in dieting patterns have shown that non-genetic factors are largely responsible."

He goes on to say that studies in mice show that yo-yo dieting affects the gut microbiome. This may be the reason for the weight gain.

We can't necessarily extrapolate from animal studies to what happens in people. But if you've been a yo-yo dieter in the past, it's definitely worth checking out how to support your gut biome (see Hack 62).

Professor Spector says:

"The solution – while we await some magic supplements – is looking after your microbes as you transition back onto normal foods after a diet. In particular, you need to feed them plenty of fibre and polyphenol-rich foods which, as well as the obvious fruit and veg, include nuts, seeds, olive oil (extra virgin), coffee, dark chocolate and even a glass of red wine."

Of course, another possible explanation for the weight gain is that people give up in despair and eat more! I hope that if you fall into this category this book will give you the information and hope you need to try a different approach.

61: Fast Weight Loss

M ost experts advise gradual weight loss, arguing that you are less likely to put the weight on again if you lose weight gradually.

For example, the Mayo Clinic[107] says:

"In some situations ... faster weight loss can be safe if it's done the right way. For example, doctors might prescribe very low calorie diets for rapid weight loss if obesity is causing serious health problems. But an extreme diet such as this requires medical supervision. In addition, it can be difficult to keep this weight off."

A study[108] published in *The Lancet. Diabetes & Endocrinology* questions this.

Participants in the study were divided into two groups and placed on two different programmes:

- a 36-week gradual programme

- a 12-week rapid weight loss programme

The aim of the intervention was for participants to lose 15% of their weight. 50% of participants in the gradual weight loss group and 81% in the rapid weight loss group achieved 12·5% or more weight loss in the allocated time. These successful participants were then put on a weight maintenance diet for 144 weeks.

Around 70% of both groups regained the weight they had lost during this time. The researchers concluded:

"The rate of weight loss does not affect the proportion of weight regained within 144 weeks. These findings are not consistent with present dietary guidelines which recommend gradual over rapid weight loss, based on the belief that rapid weight loss is more quickly regained."

Another study[109] published in the *International Journal of Endocrinology and Metabolism* looked at two groups. One group was designated the rapid weight loss group, aiming to lose at least 5% in 5 weeks The other was the slow weight loss group, aiming to lose at least 5% in 15 weeks. The researchers found:

"The results of the current study showed that both protocols of rapid WL [weight loss] and slow WL caused a reduction in waist circumference, hip circumference, total body water, body fat mass, FFM [fat free mass], LBM [lean body mass], and RMR [resting metabolic rate]. Greater reduction of waist circumference, hip circumference, and FFM was seen with slow WL and greater reduction of total body water, LBM, and RMR was seen with rapid WL."

The researchers said:

"Consistent with the current study, recent findings indicate that slow weight loss, as recommended by current guidelines, worldwide, is not a priority over rapid weight loss."

A lot of the advice that weight loss should occur over time rather than be rapid does not seem to be substantiated by research. It may well be that one or the other will work for you. The question for you to establish is which one.

If you decide to try a very low calorie diet (VLCD), this should only be attempted under specialist supervision because the potential for lack of essential nutrients is significant.

62: Gut Microbiome

More and more research is showing how important our gut biome is for our health. Your gut biome is the trillions of micro-organisms that live in the digestive tract. Professor Ana Valdes[110] and research associate Amrita Vijay of the University of Nottingham (UK) say:

"The trillions of microbes inside of our gut play many very important roles in our body. Not only does this "microbiome" regulate our metabolism and help us absorb nutrients from food into the body, it can also influence whether we are lean or obese."

They cite a study from researchers from the University of Washington in the US, who found that the presence of specific "good" microbes in the gut of people dieting to lose weight affected how many pounds they were able to lose.

The two Nottingham university academics comment:

"Though the researchers have shown this link between gut microbiome and weight loss, there is still much we don't know – including needing to verify these findings in a larger group to show these bacteria are actually involved in weight loss. The study's participants were also taking part of a commercial weight loss programme. This means the group may not be representative of the general population, which is another reason why further research is needed."

Science writer Leanne Edermaniger[111] says:

"There is a lot of research that shows long-term weight gain is associated with a gut microbiome that lacks diversity — not consuming enough dietary fibre is a contributing factor to this. Luckily, by increasing your intake of rainbow foods, you can support your whole body, a healthy weight, and your gut microbes all at once."

Although we don't know for certain that changing your gut bacteria through diet will help you lose weight, we do know that the suggested changes will benefit your general health. This makes it worth doing anyway.

This change in your diet may seem daunting, so you may be wondering if you could take a supplement of the "good bacteria".

Leanne Edermaniger cautions against this approach:

"There's no such thing as a weight loss gut bacteria supplement (so please don't buy one). The fastest way to have a significant and lasting positive impact on your microbiome is to eat a healthier diet with lots of fruit and veg, and importantly, less refined sugar, artificial sweeteners, and meat.

"Basically, gut bacteria won't directly cause you to lose weight. Instead, it's the effects of their activities rippling through your body which can help lose, gain, or maintain your weight because they help determine how much energy your body absorbs, and also how hungry or full you feel."

Yet more support for following a healthy diet, rather than simply focussing on calories in.

63: Plant-Based Diets

B eing plant-based and being vegan are not the same thing. It's perfectly possible these days to be a junk food vegan, buying highly processed meals from fast food restaurants and supermarkets, all washed down with sugary drinks. This sort of diet is not going to help you to lose weight. It's important to recognise that just because a food is suitable for vegans, it doesn't make it healthy.

Being plant-based is usually taken to mean having a diet where a large proportion consists of vegetables, beans, fruits, nuts and seeds. Some people will also eat some meat, fish and dairy too, but in much smaller quantities than in general.

Dr Shireen Kassam[112], consultant haematologist who heads up the Plant-Based Nutrition Course at the University of Winchester (UK) was interviewed by the BBC. She says:

"Scientific studies that have looked at non-vegan populations over 20-30 years show those eating the most plant foods tend to put on less weight over time than those eating the most meat, dairy and egg."

So, even if you don't want to become entirely plant-based, eating lots of plant foods can reduce the tendency to put on weight as you age.

Science writer Leanne Edermaniger[113] says:

"Research has ... shown that following a natural plant-based diet reduces calorie intake, increases weight loss, and lowers metabolic markers. It also nourishes beneficial gut bacteria because plants contain lots of different prebiotic fibers.

"In a study involving type II diabetes patients, a vegan diet was shown to be more effective at controlling blood sugar levels than a usual diabetic diet. And, in the plant diet group, calorie intake was lower, which meant weight loss was more rapid. Interestingly, the beneficial bacteria that thrive on plant foods are also associated with better blood sugar control."

Once again, the importance of the microbiome for weight control is highlighted. Eating lots of plants is shown to support the good bacteria in your gut. This is beneficial for so many reasons.

The charity Veganuary reviewed scientific research[114] on vegan diets and weight loss on their website. They cite various studies, for example:

"A meta-analysis of randomised trials published in 2016 in the *Journal of General Internal Medicine,* on the effect of vegetarian diets on obesity rates, found that vegetarian diets achieved significantly greater weight loss than energy-restriction diets, and that vegan diets produced greater weight loss than vegetarian diets.

"A two year controlled trial in *Obesity* compared a moderate low fat diet to a vegan diet. The results showed that the vegans lost significantly more weight than those on the low fat diet."

Many of these studies were completed at a time when vegan fast food and supermarket dishes weren't widely available, so being vegan was likely to mean being plant-based.

Veganuary conclude by saying:

"not all vegan diets are healthy and will lead to weight loss. With so many vegan foods readily available, it is easier than ever to rely on convenience foods that are highly processed, and high in fat and sugar. A whole food plant-based diet is rich in grains, vegetables, fruits, nuts, legumes, and is the basis for a nutritious and healthy diet to fuel your body and keep you well."

This seems to sum up the situation. Being a vegan won't automatically mean that you will lose weight. Being plant-based is likely to mean your weight will be within the healthy range. Changing to a plant-based diet is likely to help you lose and keep off excess weight.

64: Antibiotics

Science writer Leanne Edermaniger[115] says:

"Dysbiosis of the gut microbiome can result from ... antibiotics. This type of medication is linked to weight gain because they disrupt the microbial communities in your gut, either by preventing and slowing bacterial growth, or killing them.

"Yet, the link between antibiotics and weight gain isn't really a secret. Industrial agriculture has known for decades that low doses of antibiotics can encourage animals destined for meat consumption to gain weight faster."

Antibiotics can induce changes in the gut microbiome that can be detected 6 months and even two years after taking them, so the message is only take antibiotics if you really need them.

If you need to take antibiotics, be aware that you also need to eat the right food to help feed the good bacteria in your gut. See Hack 62 for more on this.

65: Is Some Food Addictive?

T his question is by no means resolved among the medical and scientific community.

Some believe that it is impossible to be addicted to something we need for our survival. They also argue that food doesn't have the same effects as drugs do.

Yet the majority view is now moving towards the idea that some food can be addictive by stimulating the reward centres of the brain. But, like a drug addict, over time you need more and more of the substance to satisfy you.

Psychologist Susan Albers[116] says:

"Many of the words that people use to describe how they feel with food are very much related to addiction, such as cravings, withdrawal and feeling out of control."

Paediatrician Minati Singh[117] writes in the academic article *Frontiers of Psychology*:

"highly palatable foods activate the same brain regions of reward and pleasure that are active in drug addiction, suggesting a neuronal mechanism of food addiction leading to overeating and obesity"

Belinda Lennerz[118] (Boston Children's Hospital, USA) and Jochen K. Lennerz (Massachusetts General Hospital, USA) write in the academic journal *Clinical Chemistry*:

"Three lines of evidence support the concept of food addiction: (1) behavioral responses to certain foods are similar compared to substances of abuse; (2) food intake regulation and addiction rely on similar neurobiological circuits; (3) individuals suffering from obesity or addiction show similar neurochemical- and brain activation patterns."

Yet they go on to say that considerable debate remains around the triggering mechanism of food addiction.

They look at a variety of research that seems to suggest that the foods involved are usually highly processed foods containing either mixed macronutrients or pure high glycaemic carbohydrate foods.

They say:

"Current obesity therapy focuses on moderation of food intake and increase of physical activity ... however, at least in a subset of vulnerable individuals, high GI [glycaemic index] carbohydrates can be considered a specific trigger that can be reduced or avoided."

See Hack 37 for more on the glycaemic index.

Ferris Jabr in an article in *Scientific American* entitled *How Sugar and Fat Trick the Brain into Wanting More Food*[119].

"For some people, palatable foods invoke such a strong response in the brain's reward circuit—and so dramatically alter their biology—that willpower will rarely, if ever, be sufficient to resist eating those foods once they are around...

"In practical terms, that means never bringing fatty, supersweet foods into the house in the first place and avoiding venues that offer them whenever possible."

Not everyone needs to avoid these foods totally. But you may be one of these people who should. That can mean some difficult conversations with family and co-workers. I suggest you show them this *Scientific American* article[120]. Hopefully reading this will mean that they are more willing to help you.

66: Be Angry!

Many teenagers love junk food and will eat it to excess and turn their noses up at salads. A research project by Christopher J. Bryan[121] and others from the University of Chicago (USA) has found that a simple and brief intervention can provide lasting protection for adolescents against the harmful effects of junk food marketing.

Food marketing is deliberately designed to create positive emotional associations with junk food and to connect it with feelings of happiness and fun. The researchers went into classrooms and taught groups of students about the way junk food manufacturers try to hook consumers on addictive junk food for financial gain. Control groups were given factual information about healthy food.

The students were followed over three months. The girls ate less junk food regardless of whether they were in the experimental or control groups. For the boys the marketing expose was much more effective; they reduced their daily purchases of unhealthy drinks and snacks in the school cafeteria by 31% in that time period, compared with the control group.

Could this be used to your advantage? Educate yourself about how junk food manufacturers use packaging and advertising to suggest that eating their products will make you popular, sexy and slim. Think about the advertisements that suggest these companies really care about you and the environment. Manufacturers deliberately manipulate the food they produce to make it irresistible, even though they know the detrimental effect it may have on people's health and happiness. Look at how much money they are making and how little tax some of them pay.

In 2015 the *New York Times*[122] showed how Coca-Cola has funded millions in research to downplay the link between sugary beverages and obesity.

Isabelle Szmigin[123], Professor of Marketing, University of Birmingham (UK) says:

"McDonald's ... used the marketing slogan "It's what I eat and what I do" in their campaign to encourage children to lead more active lifestyles. The emphasis is on activity, not cutting back on calories, and sends the message "don't blame us if you get fat – go running"."

Decide that you will not let these companies manipulate you and everyone else in a way that harms your ability to manage your weight and well-being. Do you really want to buy the products of unscrupulous companies, who do not have your best interests at heart?

In the research I quote at the beginning of this hack only the boys were significantly affected by this approach. But I still think it's worth giving it a try regardless of your gender or age.

67: Can Dieting Slow Your Metabolism?

When you lose a lot of weight, you will need fewer calories to maintain your body and to carry out your daily activities. This is to be expected. Your metabolic rate is the number of calories you burn at rest, your resting metabolic rate or RMR. Adam Collins[124] and Aoife Egan of the University of Surrey (UK) say:

"The loss of lean tissue (muscle) when you diet – which burns around 15-25 calories per kilogram each day – lowers resting metabolic rate, meaning you need fewer calories than you previously did. But the body also deliberately slows down metabolism to preserve energy stores and minimise weight loss."

This adaptation is known as metabolic adaptation or adaptive thermogenesis. Dietitian Chelsey Hegge[125] describes it like this:

"To the body there is little differentiation between a response to famine or to dieting. In both cases one's metabolism slows and hormonal alterations favor a decreased energy output to balance the lower amount of calories consumed. When "energy in" decreases, "energy out" drops in response."

A study by Erin Fothergill[126] and colleagues in the research journal *Obesity* looked at participants in the US TV series "The Biggest Loser". The show features obese or overweight contestants competing to win a cash prize by losing the highest percentage of weight relative to their initial weight. The researchers studied 16 participants:

"We found that despite substantial weight regain in the 6 years following participation in "The Biggest Loser", RMR [resting metabolic rate] remained suppressed at the same average level as at the end of the weight loss competition. Mean RMR after 6 years was ~ [approximately] 500 kcal/day lower than expected based on the measured body composition changes and the increased age of the subjects."

In other words, these participants were going to have to restrict their calorie intake more in order to lose weight than if they had never taken part in the TV programme. Remember that these participants lost a lot of weight really fast – everything about their lives was dedicated to weight loss. They often did unhealthy things – like restricting fluids – in order to weigh less. This is an extreme example of weight loss, and doesn't necessarily apply to the sort of weight loss you have experienced.

The University of Surrey researchers[127] reviewed the changes that happen as a result of weight loss – a decrease in body fat, shrinking of fat cells, changes in hormone levels, etc. They concluded:

"as contradictory as it sounds, all these changes actually result in a more efficient and ultimately healthier metabolism. For example, smaller fat cells are better for our health, as over-inflated "sick" fat cells don't work as well in getting rid of surplus sugar and fat. This can lead to high levels of sugar and fat in the blood, increasing risk of insulin resistance, diabetes, and cardiovascular disease ...

"So dieting doesn't technically ruin your metabolism but rather improves it by helping it work better. But without care, this metabolic improvement can conspire against you to regain the weight, and even overshoot your original weight."

If you have lost a lot of weight, you may need to use more calories or eat fewer calories to maintain the weight than someone who has always been around that weight. This doesn't mean it's impossible to maintain your weight. It doesn't mean it's inevitable that you will regain the weight you have lost.

Thinking that you have "messed up" your metabolism, makes it more likely that you will blame any weight you regain on your metabolism rather than on what you are eating or your activity levels. Concentrate on what you can control and be clear that it is up to you to maintain the weight you have lost.

Check out Hack 61 Fast Weight Loss and Hack 70 Weight Loss Maintenance.

68: Weight Loss Plateau

This is something that all dieters dread – the point at which the weight loss stubbornly stops. It's easy to blame it on our metabolism.

Diana M Thomas (Montclair State University, USA) and colleagues constructed two mathematical models and used them to predict when a weight loss plateau would happen. They fed data from previous research on people into their models and concluded:

"An intermittent lack of diet adherence, not metabolic adaptation, is a major contributor to the frequently observed early weight-loss plateau."

In other words, it's more likely that you've relaxed what you are doing than that your body has adapted metabolically.

This is both depressing (you don't have an excuse) and hopeful (you can do something about it).

The Mayo Clinic[128] suggests if this happens you:

- "Reassess your habits ... Make sure you haven't loosened the rules, letting yourself get by with larger portions or less exercise."

- "Cut more calories. Further cut your daily calories, provided this doesn't put you below 1,200 calories."

- "Rev up your workout ... Adding exercises such as weightlifting to increase your muscle mass will help you burn more calories."

- "Pack more activity into your day... Any physical activity will help you burn more calories."

Don't blame your metabolism. Look at what you are doing to see if it has changed in any way.

69: Plateau Purposefully

I n the book *Interval Weight Loss* by Dr Nick Fuller there is a whole chapter on diet breaks.

Dr Fuller writes:

"It's a wonderful feeling to see the weight coming off on the scales, but you still need to ensure you follow the first principle of the IWL [Interval Weight Loss] plan – *You can't fight evolution* – by putting on the brakes every second month. This will allow your body to recalibrate at its new set point along the way. I can't stress this enough."

Dr Fuller is from the Boden Institute of Obesity, Nutrition, Exercise & Eating Disorders at the University's Charles Perkins Centre and the University of Sydney School of Medicine.

He explains[129]:

"My Interval Weight Loss approach encourages weight loss in small increments. The goal is to lose a small amount of weight and then to take a break, maintaining the new body weight for a period of time before losing another small amount. Rather than activating the body's fight or flight response, the body is gently challenged to redefine its baseline body weight until the final weight-loss goal is achieved."

On the website[130] of the University of Sydney he writes:

"To prevent your metabolism slowing, impose "intervals" every second month, to allow your body the rest it needs."

Dietitian Chelsey Hegge[131] agrees:

"The human body is not designed to be in a diet mode forever. One must strategically alternate caloric deficit phases as well as weight maintenance phases to decrease metabolic adaptation. Maintenance is just as important, if not more crucial than being in a deficit to provide the proper nutrition and fueling for daily activities. A person earns the right to diet, only after being at a healthy maintenance calorie level for an extended period of time."

70: Weight Loss Maintenance

M any people believe that is pointless trying to lose weight because everyone just puts it back on again.

M T McGuire[132] (University of Pittsburg, USA) and colleagues looked at this idea and found:

"A large proportion of the American population has lost ... [an amount greater than or equal to] 10% of their maximum weight and has maintained this weight loss for at least 1 y. These findings are in sharp contrast to the belief that few people succeed in long-term weight loss maintenance."

This is in contrast to the work of Traci Mann[133], professor of psychology at the University of Minnesota (USA). She and her graduate students analysed every randomised controlled trial of diets that included a follow-up of at least two years. They concluded:

"The dieters had little benefit to show for their efforts, and the non-dieters did not seem harmed by their lack of effort. In sum, it appears that weight regain is the typical long-term response to dieting, rather than the exception."

Many of the studies I cite in this book, also record people putting all or most of their weight back on.

Your own experience may be of losing weight and then putting it back on again. This can make you feel that losing weight is a horrible struggle that is just not worthwhile. You may see a bleak future where you're either overweight/obese or you are constantly having to restrict what you eat.

This may be because you've been entirely focussed on restricting calories, as the way to lose weight. This isn't surprising when magazines, newspapers and websites are full of information about calorie restriction. It may be why the statistics for long-term mainte-nance are so depressing – too many people have just focussed on how many calories they are eating. Maybe calorie restriction is not the way to long-term success.

But let's have a look at some of the research on people who manage to keep weight gain to a minimum.

Research from the University of Colorado[134] (USA) found:

"... successful weight-loss maintainers rely on physical activity to remain in energy balance (rather than chronic restriction of dietary intake) to avoid weight regain. In the study, successful weight-loss maintainers are individuals who maintain a reduced body weight of 30 pounds or more for over a year."

Adam Collins[135] and Aoife Egan of the University of Surrey (UK) say:

"Studies show exercise (or simply physical activity) may be one way to prevent weight regain, by improving our ability to maintain our weight and can potentially minimise metabolic slowing. Exercise can also help regulate appetite and fuel burning in the short term, and may make weight loss more sustainable in the long term."

The US government Centers For Disease Control[136] says:

"To maintain your weight: Work your way up to 150 minutes of moderate-intensity aerobic activity, 75 minutes of vigorous-intensity aerobic activity, or an equivalent mix of the two each week. Strong scientific evidence shows that physical activity can help you maintain your weight over time. However, the exact amount of physical activity needed to do this is not clear since it varies greatly from person to person. It's possible that you may need to do more than the equivalent of 150 minutes of moderate-intensity activity a week to maintain your weight."

Judy Kruger[137] and colleagues from the Centers for Disease Control (USA) found:

"Self-monitoring strategies such as weighing oneself, planning meals, tracking fat and calories, exercising 30 or more minutes daily, and/or adding physical activity to daily routine may be important in successful weight loss maintenance."

The US National Weight Control Registry[138] is a research group that seeks to gather information from people who have successfully lost weight and kept it off. This is defi-nitely people we want to hear from! They found that:

"Most report continuing to maintain a low calorie, low fat diet and doing high levels of activity.

- 78% eat breakfast every day.

- 75% weigh themselves at least once a week.

- 62% watch less than 10 hours of TV per week.

- 90% exercise, on average, about 1 hour per day."

Another study[139] of National Weight Control Registry participants found:

"Decreases in leisure-time physical activity, dietary restraint, and frequency of self-weighing and increases in percentage of energy intake from fat and disinhibition [lessening self-control] were associated with greater weight regain."

Professor Debra Haire-Joshu[140] says:

"Any weight gain–prevention method that is not comprehensive, multi- component and sustainable is going to have less effectiveness. The more comprehensive an effort can be, including eating and regular activity, the more effective it will be."

M T McGuire[141] (University of Pittsburgh, USA) and colleagues say this about their research:

"This study suggests that several years of successful weight maintenance increase the probability of future weight maintenance and that weight regain is due at least in part to failure to maintain behavior changes."

Other research from M L Klem[142] (also from the University of Pittsburgh, USA) agrees that it gets easier as time goes on:

"Subjects who had maintained weight losses longer used fewer weight maintenance strategies and reported that less effort was required to diet and maintain weight and that less attention was required to maintain weight."

These are the strategies that have been shown to work for long term maintenance. It is not enough just to focus on calories, you need to look at your daily activity levels. Check out Hack 45 Changing Your Attitude To Exercise if you hate exercise.

You also need to continue or start activities, such as self-weighing (see Hack 134) and eating more low glycaemic index foods (see Hack 37 Carbohydrate-Insulin Model).

71: What's Your Scream Weight?

D r Barbara Berkeley[143], author of *Refuse To Gain* advises doctors:

"Encourage the patient to set a 'Scream Weight.' This is the weight that provokes immediate action (and screaming!) when it pops up on the scale. The scream weight is set at about 8 pounds higher than the final weight achieved in order to provide a range for acceptable weight (scream weight being the top of the range). Patients should weigh themselves every day and have a plan for reduction if they close in on their scream weight. Some people will need to adjust the scream weight up after a time as they may find that their initial goal weight was too low for them."

While this is aimed at clinicians, I think this is great advice. Think about this as you lose weight, so you have a plan to help you maintain your weight.

This can be particularly helpful if you've lost and gained weight. It can help counteract the little voice telling you that working hard to lose all this weight is pointless, because you'll only put it on again.

72: Food Diaries

The Harvard Health Blog[144] says:

"A food diary can be a useful tool … It can help you understand your eating habits and patterns, and help you identify the foods — good and not-so-good — you eat on a regular basis. Research shows that for people interested in losing weight, keeping a journal can be a very effective tool to help change behavior. In one weight loss study of nearly 1,700 participants, those who kept daily food records lost twice as much weight as those who kept no records."

The blog says that you should put three things in your food diary:

What are you eating? Write down the specific food and beverage consumed and how it is prepared (baked, broiled, fried, etc.). Include any sauces, condiments, dressings, or toppings.

How much are you eating? List the amount in household measures (cups, teaspoons, tablespoons) or in ounces. If possible, it is best to weigh and measure your food. If you are away from home, do your best to estimate the portion.

When are you eating? Noting the time that you're eating can be very helpful in identifying potentially problematic times, such as late-night snacking.

Also, make a note of any other activities you are doing at the same time. Record if you are eating with other people. Write down why you are eating. Make a note of how you feel while eating and when you have finished eating.

Food diaries seem to work in two ways:

- The effort of recording reduces the amount you eat.

- The diary gives you insights that you can use to eat less or eat more healthily.

TOPS (Take Off Pounds Sensibly) Club Inc[145] says:

"Throughout our lives, we learn that eating can give us something to do, provide a pleasant social setting, help us avoid addressing unpleasant feelings, provide a reward, recall a cherished memory or alleviate stress. Take time to journal what you were feeling when you chose to eat when you weren't physically hungry."

Psychologist Amy Walters, PhD[146] says:

"Research is clear that people who write down what they eat in a daily log are more successful at losing weight. In addition, I ask patients to record information about their thoughts, feelings, and the environment to help understand their eating behaviors and identify areas for intervention."

A research study from Duke University[147] (USA) found that overweight people who tracked daily food consumption using a free smartphone app lost a significant amount of weight – an average of 5 lbs (2.2 kg) over 3 months. This was achieved without following a particular diet.

It's unclear whether journaling by hand is more effective than typing on a computer or on an app. Try both and see if one works better for you than the other.

73: Get Up To PACE

If you've tried repeatedly to lose weight, chances are that you can count calories well. You probably know how many calories are in a whole range of food and drinks. You know which foods are high calories, but maybe you still eat them.

If that's you, try thinking about PACE instead. PACE stands for Physical Activity Calorie Equivalent. There's evidence[148] that it can be more helpful than thinking about food in terms of calories.

Amanda Daley[149], Professor of Behavioural Medicine, Loughborough University (UK), writes:

"eating 230 calories in a small bar of chocolate would require about 46 minutes of walking or 23 minutes of running to burn off these calories."

The website onhealth.com[150] gives these figures for a 175 pound (80 kg) healthy man and a 140 pound (63.5 kg) healthy woman doing the exercise for one hour:

Light Activity: 300 for the man and 240 for the woman

- Cleaning house

- Office work

- Playing baseball

- Playing golf

- Moderate Activity: 460/370 calories

- Walking briskly (3.5 mph)

- Gardening

- Cycling (5.5 mph)

- Dancing

- Playing basketball

Strenuous Activity: 730/580 calories
- Jogging (9 min/mile)

- Playing football

- Swimming

Very Strenuous Activity: 920/740 calories
- Running (7 min/mile)

- Racquetball

- Skiing

Remember that these figures are guides only, but it may make you stop and think next time you reach for that high calorie snack or meal. Work out how much time you need to spend on housework or skiing to counteract it. Actually, it's probably better to do this beforehand.

So think of the food or drink that you find hardest to resist. Work out now how much activity will be needed to counteract it. Remember this will be extra activity.

74: Spices

Do you add spices and herbs to your meals because you like the taste? Well, here are more great reasons to add spices and herbs every day to what you eat.

A review of clinical trials published in the *Journal of Functional Foods*[151] looked at 30 herbs and spices and found that eight culinary herbs and spices were reported to reduce obesity indices (such as BMI and waist circumference) significantly when compared either with the beginning of the study or against a placebo. The herbs and spices were basil, cardamom, cinnamon, coriander, garlic, ginger, nigella seed and turmeric. The exact amount given in each study varied but was between 1 g and 3 g per day for a period between 4 and 16 weeks.

Penn State University (USA) researchers[152] found that adding six grams of spices to a meal high in fat and carbohydrates resulted in lower inflammation markers hours later. See Hack 90 Chronic Inflammation on why this is important.

The researchers used a blend of basil, bay leaf, black pepper, cinnamon, coriander, cumin, ginger, oregano, parsley, red pepper, rosemary, thyme and turmeric for the study.

Connie Rogers, associate professor of nutritional sciences, said:

"If spices are palatable to you, they might be a way to make a high-fat or high-carb meal more healthful ... We can't say from this study if it was one spice in particular, but this specific blend seemed to be beneficial."

She went on to say:

"Ultimately the gold standard would be to get people eating more healthfully and to lose weight and exercise, but those behavioral changes are difficult and take time ... So in the interim, we wanted to explore whether a combination of spices that people are already familiar with and could fit in a single meal could have a positive effect."

So, spruce up your spice cupboard and add them to your meals every day, but don't think this is all you need to do to eat healthily.

75: Naturally Slim Friends

E at with a naturally slim friend and watch them carefully.

They probably eat slowly. They probably chew their food well. They stop eating or loading their fork with the next mouthful while they talk.

Your slim friend may well leave a tiny piece of pizza crust or 4 peas on their plate. They're full and they stop eating.

You probably can't eat all your meals and snacks with your slim friend but copy this way of eating in your life.

76: Eating With Friends

S uzanne Higgs and Jason Thomas wrote a review article for the academic article *Current Opinion in Behavioral Sciences*[153]. They wrote:

"If we eat with someone who is eating a large amount then we are likely to model what they eat and consume more than we would eat if we were dining alone. We are also likely to eat a large amount if we eat in a group rather than eating alone. Such 'social-facilitation' of eating has been well documented with evidence from food diaries, observational and experimental studies. On the other hand, we might eat less than usual if we think that eating a small amount will create a favourable social impression. One reason why other people have such an influence on our eating is that they provide a guide or norm for appropriate behaviour.

I'm not suggesting you should give up social eating. It's really important for our well-being. Reminding yourself of the pitfalls can help reduce the problem of eating too much, when you are with friends who eat a lot. It may also be that they want to eat less, but get drawn in. You could be doing them a favour by eating less yourself, allowing them to eat less too.

77: Eating Slowly

A na M Andrade[154] and colleagues from the University of Rhode Island (USA) found that eating slowly led to a significant decrease in energy intake and a significant increase in water consumption. Despite higher energy intake upon meal completion under the quick condition, feeling of fulness were significantly lower than for the slow condition.

Another study by Dr Alexander Kokkinos[155] and colleagues of Laiko General Hospital in Athens (Greece) provides a possible explanation for the relationship between speed eating and overeating. Their research showed that the rate at which someone eats may impact the release of gut hormones that signal the brain to stop eating.

Eating slowly can be surprisingly difficult if you've always eaten quickly. My brother says he eats quickly because I used to steal his food as a child!

So maybe you need some help. Try one or more of these:

- Play calming music while you eat

- Put a post-it note on the table reminding yourself to eat slowly.

- Put your cutlery down between mouthfuls, rather than using the time while you're eating to load up your fork or spoon with the next mouthful.

Mindfulness (Hack 53) and Intuitive Eating (Hack 55) can also be helpful.

78: Use Chopsticks

O besity researcher Dr Nick Fuller[156] of The University of Sydney (Australia) advocates people sit down at the dinner table and use chopsticks for evening meals, to encourage eating more slowly.

This hack only works if you don't normally use chopsticks! If you're adept with chopsticks, change to a knife and fork if you find that more difficult.

79: Change Hands

M any of us have lots of automatic eating habits, for example, always having popcorn at the movies/cinema or always eating chocolate while watching a favourite television show. It may be difficult to change particularly if other people are involved.

Researchers[157] from the University of Southern California (USA) have found a simple way to eat less – use your less dominant hand.

Wendy Wood, Provost Professor of Psychology and Business said:

"It's not always feasible for dieters to avoid or alter the environments in which they typically overeat. More feasible, perhaps, is for dieters top [sic] actively disrupt the established patterns of how they eat through simple techniques, such as switching the hand they use to eat... Using the non-dominant hand seemed to disrupt eating habits and cause people to pay attention to what they were eating."

80: Portion Size

S erving sizes have got larger over the years. This has led to increased calorie consumption.

The American Heart Association[158] and the Robert Woods Johnson Foundation study "A Nation at Risk: Obesity in the United States" found:

- Adults today consume an average of 300 more calories per day than they did in 1985.

- Portion sizes have grown dramatically over the last 40 years.

- Americans eat out much more than they used to.

Many of us don't know what a healthy portion is. The American Herat Association[159] says:

"You may be surprised to learn these are serving sizes:

- 1 slice of bread

- ½ cup [US measuring cup] of rice or pasta (cooked)

- ¾ cup fruit juice

- 1 cup milk or yogurt

- 2 oz. [56 grams] cheese (about the size of a domino)

- 2-3 oz. [56-85 grams] meat, poultry or fish (this is about the size of a deck of cards)"

If you've been over-sizing your portions for a long time, work to bring them down to these.

Some people find a visual cue helps when eating dinner. You can buy portion control templates.

The plates are usually divided into 3 sections:

- Fruit and vegetables

- Proteins

- Carbohydrates

You may not need to use this forever, but if your portion control is adrift try it for a while to get a new habit.

There's also portion control cutlery, which may encourage you to eat less or more slowly.

81: Down Tools!

This is a simple but effective strategy. Put your fork/spoon down once you have put it in your mouth. Pick the implement up again when your mouth is empty, and you are ready to eat more.

If you're eating something like a sandwich, chocolate bar or fruit, put it down between mouthfuls if possible.

Thin people often do this automatically. The rest of us have to learn it. Remember learning new things can take time, so give yourself the time and space to make this the automatic way you eat.

That way you are likely to eat less and enjoy your food more – your stomach has time to register that it's full, which it doesn't have if you gobble your food down.

82: Get the Fullness Message

The US National Heart Blood & Lung Institute[160] says:

"Changing the way you go about eating can make it easier to eat less without feeling deprived. It takes 15 or more minutes for your brain to get the message that you've been fed. Eating slowly will help you feel satisfied. Eating lots of vegetables and fruits can make you feel fuller. Another trick is to use smaller plates so that moderate portions do not appear too small. Changing your eating schedule, or setting one, can be helpful, especially if you tend to skip, or delay, meals and overeat later."

83: Is Plate Size Important?

In the USA[161] in the 1980s the typical dinner plate was 25 cm (9.8 inches) in diameter. In the early 2000s it was 30 cms (11.8 inches). This is an increase <u>in area</u> of 44%

Does this matter?

Common sense tells us it is likely to matter. If you have a small plate that is full, it will seem that you are eating a lot more food than a larger plate that is half full but contains the same amount of food as the smaller plate.

But the research is not yet clear.

Laura König & Gareth Hollands[162] conducted a study involving 134 adults. Participants were given just pasta to eat. On average, participants ate 19 calories less from the smaller plate. This is hardly going to make a difference to how much you weigh.

But the researchers say:

"One important thing to keep in mind when interpreting this result is that we conducted our study in a laboratory setting, where people only ate one type of food and ate alone in front of a TV... This means that we can't rule out that plate size could have an effect in real-life eating situations.

"... if you're looking to eat less or lose weight, you might not want to get rid of your smaller plates immediately – they may work for some people or in some situations, and we don't have any clear evidence that they could unwittingly make people eat more."

Brian Wensink and Koert van Ittersum[163] found that when people serve themselves, they tend to fill around 70% of the plate. This suggests that plate size is important – 70% of a smaller plate is less than 70% of a bigger plate.

My own experience is that I eat less when I use a smaller plate. This would be another strategy that's worth trying to see if it makes a difference for you.

84: Plate Colour

C harles Spence[164], Professor of Experimental Psychology and University Lecturer, University of Oxford (UK) says:

"Research shows that we rate food as tasting different depending on the colour of the crockery on which it is served. We conducted an experiment at Ferran Adria's Alicia Foundation just outside Barcelona a few years ago in which we demonstrated that people would rate a pinkish strawberry mousse as tasting 7% sweeter, 13% more flavourful and 9% more enjoyable when it was served it on a white plate rather than a black plate. Meanwhile, others have demonstrated that we will eat less junk food if it is served from a red plate than from a plate of any other colour."

It may be time to get yourself a bigger range of plate and bowl colours and experiment to find what works for you.

85: Plates With A Wide Rim

Here's an easy hack to implement when you eat at home.

A study from A D McClain[165], Stanford University (USA), and colleagues looked at the effect of plate rims on participants perceptions of how much food was on the plate. They found they overestimated the diameter of food portions by 5% and the visual area of food portions by 10% on plates with wider rims compared with plates with very narrow rims.

They also found that participants overestimated the diameter of food portions by 1.5% and the visual area of food portions by 3% on plates with rim colouring compared with plates with no colouring.

It's not a world-beating way to lose weight, but it will be a small but effective part of all the other things you are doing.

86: Fresh Slate Mentality

A University of Illinois (USA) study[166] found that women who succeeded at weight loss maintenance engaged in regular exercise and said they "listened to an inner voice" that reminded them to control their portion sizes.

These dieters also adopted a "fresh-slate mentality," forgiving themselves for "slip-ups" and "bad days," and got back on track with their eating and exercise programs right away, rather than letting one lapse in judgment or willpower trigger a downward spiral.

The American Psychological Association[167] says:

"Don't obsess over "bad days" when you can't help eating more. This is often a problem for women who tend to be overly hard on themselves for losing discipline. Look at what thoughts or feelings caused you to eat more on a particular day, and how you can deal with them in ways other than binge eating. A psychologist can help you formulate an action plan for managing these uncomfortable feelings."

Registered Dietitian Anne Myers-Wright[168] says:

"Lapses (setbacks or slips) are a normal part of change. If you can learn to cope with lapses and not let them lead to relapse or "giving up" then you will improve your chances of being able to manage your weight or other dietary changes in the long term."

She goes on to say:

"What were you thinking before you lapsed? (if anything)

What happened after the lapse?

What could you do differently next time?

You may find you can plan for avoiding future lapses this way."

Do you think you can adopt a fresh slate mentality? Be gentle with yourself and recognise that sometimes you will lapse, but the secret is to accept that and just get back to healthy eating.

87: Cravings

Do you find that if you restrict what you can eat, you just crave it more? Some research[169] in the academic journal *Current Nutrition Reports* is a source of hope. The researchers concluded:

"Dieting's bad reputation for increasing food cravings is only partially true as the relationship between food restriction and craving is more complex. While short-term, selective food deprivation may indeed increase food cravings, long-term energy restriction seems to decrease food cravings, suggesting that food deprivation can also facilitate extinction of conditioned food craving responses."

In other words, you will experience more cravings initially, but in the long run – if you persist – you will experience fewer.

If you've decided to reduce or eliminate sugar from your diet, you may experience strong cravings for it. This research tells you to hang on in there and, with time, the craving will lessen.

A study in the *Journal of Health Psychology*[170] confirmed previous research showing a link between chronic stress and food cravings for specific high-calorie non-nutritious foods, resulting in an increased body mass index. If this is true for you, it will be difficult to conquer food cravings through willpower alone. See Hack 41 Stress.

The American Heart Association[171] says:

"We have all experienced food cravings – and often those cravings have to do with texture – like something creamy or crunchy. Food textures play a big role in whether we like or dislike certain foods ...Luckily, eating healthy includes foods of all sorts of textures and flavors."

On their website they divide food cravings into 5 types and suggest healthy alternatives for each category:

- Creamy

- Crunchy

- Liquid

- Squishy

- Crispy

So do check out their website, if you feel this would be helpful.

88: Urge Surfing

Cravings can be difficult to ignore, even when you use all your willpower. Giving into them makes you feel bad about yourself. You can feel weak-willed and useless. Maybe it leads to binge eating and more despair.

If this or something similar happens to you, try urge surfing. Urge surfing is a technique from Mindfulness (see Hack 53) popularized by clinical psychologist G. Alan Marlatt. It has been used for different types of addiction, including alcohol, cigarettes[172] etc.

The strategy involves picturing addictive urges as physical waves that rise in intensity, peak, and eventually crash and subside.

John Lee on the website choosehelp.com[173] says:

"By paying great attention to what a craving actually feels like, by maintaining awareness on the craving on a second-by-second basis and by avoiding passing value judgments about what you are experiencing (this is good, this is terrible, this will never end etc.) you learn to ride over waves of cravings and you rob these cravings of much of their power."

You need more detailed instructions than this! The website offers a more comprehensive explanation of what to do, as do other websites. There are also YouTube videos on urge surfing.

89: Postponing A Snack

Nicole Mead[174] of Catolica-Lisbon School of Business and Economics (Portugal) and her colleagues tested the notion that postponing consumption of an unhealthy snack to an unspecified future time would reduce the desire for, and therefore consumption of, that snack, and found that it did.

So, give it a try when you're tempted; try saying "I won't have it now" rather than "I won't eat it".

You may think this is never going to work for you. Just give it an honest try and see – it works for some people. You could be one of them.

90: Chronic Inflammation

You may be wondering why I've included research on inflammation in a book about weight loss. Let me explain. There is a clear link between obesity and chronic inflammation.

People are often unaware that they are suffering from chronic inflammation. They may only recognise inflammation as an acute symptom – a sore throat or an infected cut. Chronic inflammation is often hidden, although you may experience joint stiffness, for example.

Mohammed S. Ellulu[175] (Universiti Putra, Malysia) and colleagues explain in the journal *Archives Of Medical Science* that obesity predisposes you to be in a pro-inflammatory state via increase in inflammatory body biochemicals. These include interleukin-6 and tumour necrosis factor alpha. There are also reduced levels of the hormone adiponectin, which has a completely anti-inflammatory function in the body. Chronic inflammation of the body has been linked to heart disease, strokes, type 2 diabetes and certain cancers. The same diseases have been linked to obesity. Other illnesses such as arthritis and psoriasis are linked to chronic inflammation too.

So, obesity appears to increase chronic inflammation in the body. It is thought that this is the mechanism that links obesity and chronic diseases together. Reducing inflammation in the body is likely to be beneficial for health.

Chronic inflammation may also be a contributory factor to obesity, as well as being a result of obesity. An article in *Circulatory Review*[176] says:

"Inflammation, particularly long-term chronic inflammation, may play important roles in the development and progression of obesity-linked insulin resistance and T2DM [type 2 diabetes mellitus] through multiple pathways regulating metabolism. Reduction or inhibition of inflammation is mostly associated with improvements in insulin resistance and metabolic functions in animal models of obesity and therefore holds promise as a new therapy for obesity-linked metabolic disease."

Harvard T H Chan School of Public Health[177] (USA) explains it like this:

"Fat cells, especially those stored around the waist, secrete hormones and other substances that fire inflammation. Although inflammation is an essential component of the immune system and part of the healing process, inappropriate inflammation causes a variety of health problems. Inflammation can make the body less responsive to insulin and change the way the body metabolizes fats and carbohydrates, leading to higher blood sugar levels and, eventually, to diabetes and its many complications."

So, you now may be convinced that it's important to consider chronic inflammation, but what to do about it?

Losing weight will reduce the link between obesity and chronic diseases for most people. Also look at Hack 74 on spices.

There are many aspects to reducing the chronic inflammation that may be contributing to you becoming obese. These include reducing your stress levels (see Hack 41), limiting processed foods and eating a healthy diet with nuts, fruit and veggies. Stopping smoking and reducing alcohol consumption are also helpful in reducing inflammation.

There is a lot we still do not know about the role of chronic inflammation in the body but working to reduce the levels can only be beneficial for you in the long term.

91: Sit At A Table

D on't eat standing up - this is usually a sign you are rushing your food and not paying attention to what you are eating. If you do this, you're likely to eat more food than you need. Sit down even if you are "just" snacking.

Sit at the table to eat, but clear the table of bills, things to do, etc. It doesn't help you to control what you eat if you're looking at unpaid bills.

Nutritionist and health writer Conner Middelmann describes the strategy like this in *Psychology Today*[178]:

"Do you want to know about a diet that requires neither calorie-counting nor deprivation and doesn't involve weight-loss books, punishing exercise routines or expensive supplements? It's free, it's simple and anyone can do it. In fact, there's only one simple rule to follow: you may only eat when you are sitting down. Not in a car, not at a desk or in a subway train, but at a table designed for the consumption of food. Let's call it the Sit-Down Diet."

92: Peppermint & Cravings

C lean your teeth whenever you get cravings. It can help. Preferably use a really strong toothpaste.

The Heart Research Institute UK[179] says:

"Peppermint is actually an appetite suppressant, and if you brush your teeth immediately after eating, it will help take away the desire to nibble on food in the hours after. Chewing gum has the same effect. Brushing teeth is also great for healthy teeth and gums."

When you've finished your evening meal, clean your teeth with a strong peppermint flavoured toothpaste.

93: Weight Loss & Happiness

M any people want to lose weight because they think it will make them happier, but does it?

Do a reality check. Weighing ten pounds (five kilos) less is probably not going to make you deliriously happy, except in the short run. You'll still have money problems or work problems or other trials and tribulations that will need sorting out.

Recognise that losing weight and eating more healthily is not going to be completely plain sailing. You will make mistakes, but that doesn't make you a bad person or mean that you will fail in the long run. Don't set yourself unrealistic targets – it probably took you a long time to weigh this much. Be patient with yourself.

There's evidence that if we're happy, it's easier to lose weight. Caroline Rushforth, an NLP coach explains it succinctly (www.mindbodygreen.com[180]):

"I realized the main culprit in my battle with weight had always been my thinking and my habits. I needed to work on my self esteem, self acceptance, and happiness in my own skin. I thought losing weight would give me those qualities, but in reality, I had to develop them before I could lose the weight."

So, rather than waiting to be happy once you've lost the weight, or pinning future happiness on a new, slimmer you, start focussing on being happier right now.

94: Stand Backwards

All-you-can eat buffets can be a nightmare if you're struggling to control the amount you eat. Deciding beforehand how much to eat and reminding yourself about your goals can just fly out of the window when faced with tasty treats.

One simple strategy may help. Stand or sit with your back to the buffet, so that you're not constantly looking at all that tempting food.

This won't solve the problem entirely, but it may lessen how much you end up eating.

95: Negative-Calorie Foods

A negative calorie food would require the body to use more calories digesting than the food contains. This sounds like a dream food for dieters.

The US Academy of Nutrition and Dietetics[181] says:

"... the claim that celery, lettuce or other fruits and vegetables take more energy to chew and digest than they actually contain, is based on wishful thinking and not research. Although many vegetables and fruits may be low in calories or provide a good source of dietary fiber, make no mistake, they still count towards a day's intake and aren't actually a "negative calorie" food."

96: Emotional Eating

S haron A. Suh, Ph.D.[182] writes on her blog:

"Notice what you are eating and what is eating you."

She goes on to say:

You might ... consider rating your emotional satisfaction during and after eating on a scale of 1 to 5, with 1 being not satisfied at all and 5 being completely satisfied. You might find some new insights about the level of satisfaction in relation to the level of volume, and you might begin to trust your body's wisdom and ability to inform you when you are hungry, full, and satisfied. Remember—all food is medicine and finding the right dose for yourself is one of the first steps toward becoming a mindful eater."

Helpguide.org[183] offers this handy way to help you distinguish between emotional hunger and physical hunger:

EMOTIONAL HUNGER	PHYSICAL HUNGER
Comes on suddenly	Comes on gradually
Feels like it needs to be satisfied instantly	Can wait
Craves specific comfort foods	Open to options – lots of things sound good
Isn't satisfied with a full stomach	Stops when you are full
Triggers feelings of guilt, powerlessness and shame	Doesn't make you feel bad about yourself.

The website goes on to say:

"Eating can be a way to temporarily silence or "stuff down" uncomfortable emotions, including anger, fear, sadness, anxiety, loneliness, resentment, and shame. While you're numbing yourself with food, you can avoid the difficult emotions you'd rather not feel.

"If you don't know how to manage your emotions in a way that doesn't involve food, you won't be able to control your eating habits for very long. Diets so often fail because they offer logical nutritional advice which only works if you have conscious control over your eating habits. It doesn't work when emotions hijack the process, demanding an immediate payoff with food.

"In order to stop emotional eating, you have to find other ways to fulfill yourself emotionally. It's not enough to understand the cycle of emotional eating or even to understand your triggers, although that's a huge first step. You need alternatives to food that you can turn to for emotional fulfillment."

Wise words. If you feel they apply to you, it may be time to seek help through counselling or other therapies.

97: Intermittent Fasting

Intermittent fasting (IF) is usually divided into 3 categories:

- Time-restricted feeding: eating only during a certain number of hours each day.

- Alternate day fasting: alternating between eating whatever you want on one day and fasting the next day with reduced or no calories.

- Periodic fasting or whole-day fasting: the 5:2 diet where there are one or two fasting days per week is an example of this. During the fasting days, consumption of approximately 500 to 700 calories, or about 25% of regular daily caloric intake, may be allowed instead of complete fasting.

A review of over 25 research studies was conducted by Professor Krista Varady[184] of the University of Illinois (USA). She and her colleagues studied research involving three types of intermittent fasting:

- Alternate day fasting, which typically involves a feast day alternated with a fast day where 500 calories are consumed in one meal.

- 5:2 diet, a modified version of alternate day fasting that involves five feast days and two fast days per week.

- Time-restricted eating, which confines eating to a specified number of hours per day, usually four to 10 hours, with no calorie restrictions during the eating period.

She said:

"We noted that intermittent fasting is not better than regular dieting; both produce the same amount of weight loss and similar changes in blood pressure, cholesterol and inflammation."

A study published by Ruth Schübel[185] and colleagues in the *American Journal Of Clinical Nutrition* looked at the results for two groups – one restricting calories generally and the other restricting calories intermittently. The study lasted for 50 weeks. The researchers concluded:

"Our results on the effects of the "5:2 diet" indicate that ICR [intermittent calorie restriction] may be equivalent but not superior to CCR [continuous calorie restriction] for weight reduction and prevention of metabolic diseases."

Researchers led by Dr Jonathan Johnston[186] from the University of Surrey (UK) investigated the impact changing mealtimes has on dietary intake, body composition and blood risk markers for diabetes and heart disease.

Participants were split into two groups – those who were required to delay their breakfast by 90 minutes and have their dinner 90 minutes earlier, and those who ate meals as they would normally (the controls). Participants were required to provide blood samples and complete diet diaries before and during the 10-week intervention and complete a feedback questionnaire immediately after the study. Participants were not asked to stick to a strict diet. They could eat freely, provided it was within a certain eating window.

The researchers found that those who changed their mealtimes lost on average more than twice as much body fat as those in the control group, who ate their meals as normal.

57% of participants noted a reduction in food intake either due to reduced appetite, decreased eating opportunities or a cutback in snacking (particularly in the evenings). It is currently uncertain whether the longer fasting period undertaken by this group was also a contributing factor to this reduction in body fat.

43% of the participants felt they would not be able to maintain the changed eating times because it didn't fit in with their family and social life.

If you could do this without disrupting your family/work life, this is definitely something that is worth considering.

Melina Jampolis[187], M.D., is a board-certified physician nutrition specialist, specialising in nutrition for weight loss and disease prevention. She thinks intermittent fasting is hard for most people:

"Most people are talking about time-restricted eating, which is eating in a six to eight-hour window and then fasting the remainder of the day. This is nuanced, though. Studies have shown that the window is just as important. All of the research has been done from 10 a.m. to 6 p.m. And that really is the rub.

"It's easy to skip breakfast. But for a lot of people, it's really not that livable to stop eating at 6 p.m. You're sitting there at the end of the day, you're relaxing, you're watching TV—and you're just going to drink chamomile tea? But that's where the research is the most robust."

Khara Lucius[188], a naturopathic doctor from the University of Pittsburg (USA) disagrees. She says:

"One of the advantages of IF is that it allows the individual to focus less on what they are eating, and rather on when they are eating. This flexible approach may be more appealing to many individuals, more sustainable, and often increases patient satisfaction. In addition, patients can be provided with information on the findings relevant to the different forms of IF, and may have a degree of choice with regard to which regimen they would prefer or find most realistic based on their own lifestyle factors."

So, the research evidence is not yet clear about whether intermittent fasting is beneficial for long term weight loss. Some people clearly find it inconvenient and disruptive, whereas others find it helpful. So, this one is over to you to decide.

98: Sugar or Fat

For many years there has been an emphasis on low-fat foods for people who want to lose weight. We were told that if we wanted to lose weight, we should eat low-fat foods. Many products in supermarkets were promoted as low-fat alternatives to the regular product.

Yet the science behind this is far from what it should be. In the 1960s, the sugar industry funded research that downplayed the risks of sugar and highlighted the hazards of fat. They turned the focus of scientists, dietitians and the public away from sugar and pointed the finger at fat in the diet.

A study published in the prestigious *New England Journal of Medicine*[189] in 1967 did not disclose that it was funded by the sugar industry. It suggested there were major problems with all the studies that implicated sugar in coronary heart disease. It concluded that cutting fat out of American diets was the best way to address coronary heart disease.

From this start a whole industry was built focusing on how bad fat was for you. Many dieters misguidedly believed that cutting fat intake as close to zero as possible would be hugely beneficial.

You do not need to eat sugar in order to be healthy, but you do need to eat healthy fats. See Hack 101 Low Fat Diets for more about this.

99: Sugar Detox

Going on a "sugar detox" seems like a great decision for weight control and your overall health. But it depends on what you mean by a sugar detox.

It definitely means excluding or minimising refined sugar. Refined sugar is produced in many forms including sucrose crystals and high-fructose corn syrup.

These are found most obviously in baked goods, confectionery, chocolate and sweetened drinks. It's also the sugar crystals (brown or white) that you may put in hot drinks or on your breakfast cereals. But refined sugar is also found in a whole range of other foods, such as canned vegetables, pasta sauces and many breakfast cereals.

Jennifer Rooke[190], Assistant Professor of Community Health & Preventive Medicine, Morehouse School of Medicine (USA) explains:

"Refined sugars are not directly toxic to cells, but they can combine with proteins and fats in food and in the bloodstream to produce toxic substances such as advanced glycation end products (AGEs). High blood glucose levels may produce glycated low-density lipoproteins. High levels of these and other glucose-related toxic substances are associated with an increased risk of a wide range of chronic health problems, including cardiovascular disease and diabetes."

So, a sugar detox that excludes or dramatically reduces refined sugar is definitely beneficial for your health and probably what you weigh too. Better still if you stick to it long-term, rather than just seeing it as a temporary thing to do.

So far, so good. But what about other sources of sugar such as fruit?

Assistant professor Rooke says:

"Humans evolved to crave sweet tastes to get the nutrients needed to survive. A daily supply of vitamins, minerals and fiber is needed because our bodies cannot make them. The best source of these substances for our ancient ancestors was sweet, ripe, delicious fruit. In addition, fruits contain phytonutrients and antioxidants, chemicals produced only by plants."

This type of sugar is beneficial for us, because it comes packaged with all these other goodies. Fruit should form part of a healthy diet. Sucrose and high-fructose corn syrup are often described as empty calories, because they don't contain all these valuable nutrients.

Assistant professor Rooke concludes her review article, published in *The Conversation*[191] with this:

"Eliminating foods sweetened with refined sugar is a worthy goal. But don't think of it as a "detox" – it should be a permanent lifestyle change. The safest way to go on a refined sugar "detox" is to increase your intake of nutrient-dense fruits and vegetables. Once you eliminate refined sugar, you'll likely find that your taste buds become more sensitive to – and appreciative of – the natural sweetness of fruits."

You may be wondering about brown sugar. Yes, it does contain some minerals that white sugar doesn't contain. But the quantity is so insignificant it doesn't justify the sugar that goes with it.

You may also be wondering about fruit juice – the sort that is only fruit and doesn't contain any added sugar. The problem with fruit juice is that it doesn't contain the same level of nutrients as the whole fruit. In particular there is less fibre. In general, most authorities advise consuming only one glass of fruit juice a day.

So, by all means eliminate or massively reduce sugar in your diet. But keep some fruit in it for all the beneficial effects that it brings.

100: Low Carb Diets

Carbohydrates are starches, sugars, and fibre found in grains bread, pasta, rice, cookies, vegetables, fruit, and milk products. Low carb diets have become very popular for weight loss. The keto diet (or ketogenic diet) is an extreme version of this.

The idea behind the keto diet is that low levels of carbohydrates and very high levels of fat and protein will force the body to use fat as fuel, resulting in weight loss.

Sophie Medlin[192], Lecturer in Nutrition and Dietetics, King's College London (UK) says:

"Most people calling their diet a keto diet are simply following a low or very low carbohydrate diet. Low carbohydrate diets can be helpful, at least in the short term, for some people to lose weight. However, as with the true ketogenic diet, most people can't stick with a very low carbohydrate diet for long."

Even if people can stick to it, is it effective?

A review[193] of randomised controlled trials lasting one to two years found that the average difference in weight-loss between those on low-carb versus balanced carb diets was just under one kilogram (approximately 2 lb).

Also, many researchers think it is a diet that is not healthy in the long term.

Jennifer Rooke[194], Assistant Professor of Community Health & Preventive Medicine, Morehouse School of Medicine (USA) cautions:

"Low-carb diets may lead to weight loss, but at the expense of health. Diets that significantly reduce carbohydrates are associated with nutrient deficiencies and higher risk of death from any cause. On low-carbohydrate ketogenic diets the body will break down muscles and turn their protein into glucose. The lack of fiber causes constipation."

The Harvard T H Chan School of Public Health[195] (USA) says:

"Possible symptoms of extreme carbohydrate restriction that may last days to weeks include hunger, fatigue, low mood, irritability, constipation, headaches, and brain "fog.""

Though these uncomfortable feelings may subside, staying satisfied with the limited variety of foods available and being restricted from otherwise enjoyable foods like a crunchy apple or creamy sweet potato may present new challenges.

"Some negative side effects of a long-term ketogenic diet have been suggested, including increased risk of kidney stones and osteoporosis, and increased blood levels of uric acid (a risk factor for gout). Possible nutrient deficiencies may arise if a variety of recommended foods on the ketogenic diet are not included... Because whole food groups are excluded, assistance from a registered dietitian may be beneficial in creating a ketogenic diet that minimizes nutrient deficiencies."

The Heart Research Institute UK[196] also believes a health professional should be involved:

"A ketogenic diet is very low in carbohydrate (less than 10 per cent of energy coming from carbohydrates) and it requires the elimination of a range of healthy whole-food groups ... The removal of these foods can have implications for gut health, nutrient deficiency and metabolic health, which is why it's important to consult with a healthcare professional before commencing a restrictive dietary pattern."

Harvard T H Chan School of Public Health[197] (USA) says:

"Foods high in carbohydrates are an important part of a healthy diet ... But carbohydrate quality is important ... The healthiest sources of carbohydrates - unprocessed or minimally processed whole grains, vegetables, fruits and beans - promote good health by delivering vitamins, minerals, fiber, and a host of important phytonutrients."

If you follow a low carb diet and are feeling much better, it may be simply because you are cutting out highly processed food. Most research suggests you are better focussing on eating some healthy carbs for your long-term health, and that low carb diets aren't particularly effective in the long-term.

Clare Collins[198], Laureate Professor in Nutrition and Dietetics, and colleagues from the University of Newcastle (UK) says:

"Ultimately, if you love carbs and want to lose weight, you can. Plan to lower your kilojoule and carb intake by not eating ultra-processed, energy-dense, nutrient-poor (junk) foods, while still eating carbohydrates from healthy foods."

101: Low Fat Diets

The Harvard T H Chan School Of Public Health[199] (USA) says:

"... research has shown that low-fat diets are ineffective, and moreover, that eating healthy fats is beneficial for health."

They go on to say:

"In the eight-year Women's Health Initiative Dietary Modification Trial, women assigned to a low-fat diet didn't lose or gain more weight than women eating their usual fare."

Walter C Willett[200] and Rudolph L Leibel argue in the *American Journal Of Medicine*:

"within the United States, a substantial decline in the percentage of energy from fat during the last 2 decades has corresponded with a massive increase in the prevalence of obesity. Diets high in fat do not appear to be the primary cause of the high prevalence of excess body fat in our society, and reductions in fat will not be a solution."

The Harvard Health Blog[201] says:

"... don't be afraid to go back to fat. Just make sure it's the healthy fats like avocado, olive oil, and nuts. Don't cut out the fat, and don't make a habit of eating products labeled "fat free.""

Melina Jampolis[202], M.D., is a board-certified physician nutrition specialist, specialising in nutrition for weight loss and disease prevention. She says:

"You need healthy fat to absorb the fat-soluble nutrients in fruits and vegetables. You need it for satiety. So I don't tell people to cut fat. But never eat fat alone. Always combine it with a lower calorie density food. If you think like that and get in the habit of doing that, you will be more mindlessly able to manage your weight and optimize your health."

So, the hack here is not to try a low-fat diet to lose weight! Of course, this doesn't mean you should eat lots of fat, but a diet strategy that simply focusses on eliminating fats as much as possible is almost certainly not the way to go.

102: Nuts & Weight

D o you think that nuts should be excluded from your diet, as they are so high calorie? Well, think again. Research is showing that nuts eaten in moderation are actually beneficial for weight loss, as well as having a whole host of other health benefits.

Researchers[203] analysed US data from three longitudinal studies of health professionals - Health Professionals Follow-up Study, 1986 to 2010, Nurses' Health Study, 1986 to 2010 and the Nurses' Health Study II, 1991 to 2011. Their results were published in the *BMJ Nutrition, Prevention & Health*. They concluded that:

"... increasing daily consumption of nuts is associated with less long-term weight gain and a lower risk of obesity in adults. Replacing 0.5 servings/day of less healthful foods with nuts may be a simple strategy to help prevent gradual long-term weight gain and obesity."

A half serving of nuts would be 14 gms/0.5 ounces.

Another study published in the *European Journal of Nutrition*[204] came to a similar conclusion. Peanuts, which are technically a groundnut, were included in the study along with almonds, hazelnuts, pistachios and walnuts.

The researchers found that participants gained a mean average of 2.1 kilograms during the five-year period of the study. However, participants who ate the most nuts not only had less weight gain than the nut-abstaining people, but they also enjoyed a 5 percent lower risk of becoming overweight or obese.

The lead researcher was Joan Sabaté, MD, DrPH, director of the Center for Nutrition, Lifestyle and Disease Prevention at Loma Linda University Adventist Health Sciences Center (USA). He said:

"Eat nuts during your meal ... Put them at the center of your plate to replace animal products. They're very satiating [filling/satisfying]."

Personally, I love nuts. It's great to know that eating them also benefits my health.

103: High Protein Diets

O liver Witard[205], Lecturer in Health & Exercise Science, University of Stirling
(Scotland) says:

"High-protein diets are ... widely recognised to control food intake by making you feel
fuller for longer compared with high carbohydrate or fat foods. This helps explain why
such diets have been shown to help reduce weight regain following weight loss.

"High-protein diets are also linked to greater weight loss from fat mass and the preser-
vation of muscle. Several scientific studies in overweight/obese women have examined
weight-loss diets that include around 30% of total daily energy intake from protein. The
studies found that these high-protein diets were more likely to direct weight loss to fat
mass and away from muscle, particularly when combined with exercise training."

He recognises that some researchers have highlighted possible health problems of a
long-term high protein diet but concludes:

"High-protein diets, irrespective of food or supplement source, do effectively promote
weight loss and the health concerns surrounding these diets are not well founded."

Jaecheol Moon[206] (National University Hospital, Korea) and Jaecheol Moon (National University School of Medicine, Korea) agree. Writing in the *Journal Of Obesity
And Metabolic Syndrome* they say:"Clinical trials with various designs have found that
HPD [high protein diet] induces weight loss and lowers cardiovascular disease risk factors
such as blood triglycerides and blood pressure while preserving FFM [fat-free mass] ...
Contrary to some concerns, there is no evidence that HPD is harmful to the bones or
kidneys. However, longer clinical trials that span more than one year are required to
examine the effects and safety of HPD in more depth."

Researchers[207] at Washington University School of Medicine (USA) did find a problem when looking at post-menopausal women. One of the benefits of weight loss is an
improvement in insulin sensitivity, which is critical to lowering diabetes risk. They did

not find this occurred in the women following a high protein diet, even though they lost weight.

The participants were randomly placed into one of three groups for the 28-week study. In the control group, women were asked to maintain their weight. In another group, the women ate a weight-loss diet that included the recommended daily allowance (RDA) of protein: 0.8 grams per kilogram of body weight. For a 55-year-old woman who weighs 180 pounds, that would come to about 65 grams of protein per day.

In the third group, the women ate a diet designed to help lose weight, but they consumed more protein, taking in 1.2 grams per kilogram of body weight, or almost 100 grams for that same 180-pound woman.

The researchers focused on protein because there is a common belief that, if post-menopausal women consume extra protein, it will help preserve lean tissue, keeping them from losing too much muscle while they lose fat.

Professor Bettina Mittendorfer. the lead researcher, said:

"The women who ate more protein did tend to lose a little bit less lean tissue, but the total difference was only about a pound. We question whether there's a significant clinical benefit to such a small difference."

The research is not at a stage where we can say for certainty that long-term use of a high protein diet does not carry a health risk for some people. It certainly seems that the evidence is mounting that a diet with more protein may help with weight loss.

104: Fill Up On Fibre

F ibre doesn't contain any nutrients, but it is an important part of your diet. It helps you feel full, is food for your gut bacteria and helps prevent constipation. Fibre can also help weight control.

Foods that are high in fibre include wholemeal bread, brown rice, fruit, vegetables and legumes/beans.

A research article in *The Journal of Nutrition*[208] concluded:

"Dietary fiber intake, independently of macronutrient and caloric intake, promotes weight loss and dietary adherence in adults with overweight or obesity consuming a calorie-restricted diet."

Some dietary recommendations are quite complex. A study published in the Annals of Internal Medicine[209] compared a diet based on the dietary recommendation of the American Heart Association (AHA) with a single dietary change – an increase of fibre in the diet.

"The more complex AHA diet may result in up to 1.7 kg more weight loss [over one year]; however, a simplified approach to weight reduction emphasizing only increased fiber intake may be a reasonable alternative for persons with difficulty adhering to more complicated diet regimens."

If you're someone who likes to keep things simple, going for this one change may be beneficial. Also check out Hack 05 Keep It Simple.

Eating more fibre doesn't mean just eating more wholemeal bread. It also means eating more fruit, vegetables and legumes/beans.

The British Nutrition Foundation[210] suggests:

- Choose a high fibre breakfast cereal e.g. wholegrain cereal like wholewheat biscuit cereal, no added sugar muesli, bran flakes or porridge. Why not add some fresh fruit, dried fruit, seeds and/or nuts?

- Go for wholemeal or seeded wholegrain breads. If your family only typically likes white bread, why not try the versions that combine white and wholemeal flours as a start.

- Choose wholegrains like wholewheat pasta, bulgur wheat or brown rice.

- Go for potatoes with skins e.g. baked potato, wedges or boiled new potatoes – you can eat these hot or use for a salad.

- For snacks try fruit, vegetable sticks, rye crackers, oatcakes, unsalted nuts or seeds.

- Include plenty of vegetables with meals – either as a side dish/salad or added to sauces, stews or curries – this is a good way of getting children to eat more veg.

- Keep a supply of frozen vegetables so you are never without.

- Add pulses like beans, lentils or chickpeas to stews, curries and salads.

- Have some fresh or fruit canned in natural juice for dessert or a snack.

You may be concerned about wind/gas if you increase your fibre intake. Producing a lot of gas can be embarrassing and painful. The gas occurs because bacteria within the colon produce gas as a by-product of their digestion of fibre.

Harvard Health[211] say:

"... be careful about eating a lot of fiber at once. Overdoing it can cause gas, bloating, diarrhea, and abdominal cramps as your gut bacteria try to process all the new fiber. These problems go away after a while as your digestive system gets used to the higher fiber levels, but you can avoid them by adding extra fiber gradually to your diet. For example, try to add just one more serving of a high-fiber food to your daily diet for a week, then see how your body feels. Give yourself another week, if needed. If everything is okay, add another daily serving for a week. Continue this pattern until you reach your daily quota of fiber.

"Also, make sure to drink plenty of fluids each day—about 16 ounces of water, four times a day. Increasing the water you drink can help fiber pass through your digestive system and avoid stomach distress."

Coral Sirett of Zest Health has written a very interesting article entitled *15 Ways With Pulses*[212]. She says:

"If you have been put off eating more beans because you're concerned about wind [gas] my advice is to increase the amount you eat gradually. This will help your body to adjust to the increase in fibre.

"You can also make pulses more digestible by rinsing them if you buy canned. The easiest beans to digest are black-eyed peas, adzuki, lentils and mung beans. You may also find them easier to digest if you eat with another source of protein such as quinoa, rice or barley."

105: Magic Pills

The National Institutes Of Health[213] (USA) says:

"there's little scientific evidence that weight-loss supplements work. Many are expensive, some can interact or interfere with medications, and a few might be harmful."

Dr Joe Schwarcz[214] of McGill University (Canada) says:

"It is unbelievable what people will believe. Especially when it comes to weight loss. No matter how many "magic" pills have come and gone, hope reigns eternal that the next one that comes around will deliver the miracle of melting away the fat without paying attention to calories or energy expenditure."

I think this is harsh. Many people are desperate to lose weight. They have tried and failed many times. All that seems left as an option is some magical ingredient that will do the job.

I hope this book will give you some alternative strategies to try. They may not be magic solutions, but that's probably true of all those weight loss supplements too.

There is one possible exception to what I have said and that is in Hack 178 Alpha-Lipoic Acid and Hack 31 Omega 3 Fatty Acids.

106: Celebrities

C elebrities and influencers often showcase a fabulous lifestyle and enviable bodies. They may explain how they do it, but they often don't reveal all the professionals who work hard behind the scenes to make them look this good.

Dr Nick Fuller[215], from the Boden Institute of Obesity, Nutrition, Exercise & Eating Disorders at the University of Sydney School of Medicine (Australia) says:

"Diets have only contributed to the very problem they claim to solve – the obesity epidemic – and we largely have social media to blame ... These days it seems like everyone is a so-called wellness and weight loss expert. But obesity needs to be treated seriously, and advice should be given by people qualified to do so.

"These 'influencers' and celebrities we follow on Instagram generally don't know what they are talking about, and their advice or programs are typically not evidence based – it's anecdata."

107: Weekend Eating

There are two schools of thoughts about what to do at weekends, when you are dieting. Some people say it works best if you ease up over the weekend. Others say consistency is the key, so you carry on through the weekend.

Rui Jorge[216] and colleagues from the University of Lisbon (Portugal) say:

"On the one hand, a more flexible dietary pattern on weekends and holidays may reduce boredom, which can precipitate dieting lapses, and allow a more realistic journey from a long-term perspective. On the other hand, being more flexible may increase exposure to high-risk situations, creating more opportunity for loss of control...

"Adopting a less strict diet regimen during weekends, when compared to weekdays, was a behavioral strategy associated with long-term weight management in our sample of previously successful weight loss maintainers. Advising a stricter dietary approach during the weekend, when compared to weekdays, can be counterproductive and should be avoided in those trying to maintain their weight loss."

A A Gorin[217] and colleagues of Brown University (USA) came to a similar conclusion:

"Participants who reported a consistent diet across the week were 1.5 times more likely to maintain their weight within 5 pounds over the subsequent year ... than participants who dieted more strictly on weekdays."

These two studies found opposing results. The Lisbon study found that people did better if they were less strict at the weekends, whereas the US study found that maintaining the same strategy the whole week worked better! The difference could be down to cultural differences or something in the design of the studies that isn't immediately obvious.

Both these studies were looking at people who had successfully lost weight and were now long-term weight maintainers, so this doesn't necessarily apply while you are trying to lose weight.

A study by Susan B. Racette[218] and colleagues of Washington University School of Medicine, USA, found that eating more rather than exercising less was the main factor in weight gain or stopping weight loss.

If you have been gradually putting on weight over the years, it may well be you need to look at what you are eating most weekends if you want to stop the gain.

If you're struggling to lose weight, take a closer look at what you eat over the weekend. This could be the key to getting back on track.

108: Metabolic Confusion Diet

Adam Collins[219], Senior Teaching Fellow, Nutrition, University of Surrey (UK) describes this diet as

"... one of the latest fad diets to be blowing up on social media. Like many fad diets, it promises you can lose weight while still eating what you want.

"Fans of the diet claim that by switching between very low-calorie days and high calorie days, you can lose weight while simultaneously speeding up your metabolism. It may sound promising, but there's no research to back these claims."

Adam Collins goes on to say:

"... while these diets may be successful in getting people to eat less, they may actually reinforce bad eating habits and poor diet quality (such as consuming high-energy, highly-processed foods and drinks), as people may think they can "treat" themselves following low-calorie days. Indeed, research has shown people following these diets have a less nutritious diet than those following traditional calorie-controlled diets."

There is no evidence that the metabolic confusion diet slows the body's adaption to weight loss.

For more on this see Hack 67 Can Dieting Slow Your Metabolism?

109: Paleo Diet

A paleo diet is based on foods similar to what might have been eaten during the Paleolithic era, from approximately 2.5 million to 10,000 years ago. This is the time when humans were hunter gatherers.

It usually includes lean meats, fish, fruits, vegetables, nuts and seeds. It limits foods, such as dairy products, legumes and grains, that became common when humans started farming.

There have been criticisms of the theory of the paleo diet, including disagreement about what food existed at the time and how closely it resembles modern food.

The Harvard T H Chan School of Public Health[220] (USA) says:

"Some randomized controlled trials have shown the Paleo diet to produce greater short-term benefits than diets based on national nutrition guidelines, including greater weight loss, reduced waist circumference, decreased blood pressure, increased insulin sensitivity, and improved cholesterol. However these studies were of short duration (6 months or less) with a small number of participants (less than 40)."

One larger randomized controlled trial[221] followed 70 post-menopausal Swedish women with obesity for two years. The women were placed on either a Paleo diet or a Nordic Nutrition Recommendations (NNR) diet. Both groups significantly decreased fat mass and weight circumference at 6 and 24 months. The paleo diet produced greater fat loss at 6 months, but not at 24 months.

Apart from whether the paleo diet is effective for long term weight management, it's important to consider if it is a healthy diet.

Researchers[222] from Edith Cowan University (Australia) compared 44 people on the diet with 47 following a traditional Australian diet. They found that the people who follow the paleo diet have twice the amount of a key blood biomarker linked closely to heart disease. In other words, people following a paleo diet are more susceptible to heart disease.

Associate Professor Sof Andrikopoulos[223] of University of Melbourne (Australia) says that based on his research this type of diet is not recommended. He says this is particularly true for people who are already overweight and lead sedentary lifestyles.

He says mass media hype around these diets, particularly driven by celebrity chefs, celebrity weight-loss stories in the tabloid media and reality TV shows, are leading to more people trying fad diets backed by little evidence. In people with pre-diabetes or diabetes, the low-carb, high-fat (LCHF) diet could be particularly risky, he said.

110: Flexible Dieting

Flexible dieting has two meanings. It can just mean that someone follows a weight loss diet that doesn't exclude any foods, or it can mean a diet that "tracks macros" (carbohydrates, fat and protein).

Both are more flexible than strict calorie counting with excluded foods. There have been some studies[224] that have shown that rigid dieting is more likely to be associated with eating disorders, but it is difficult to establish which comes first. Are people who are likely to suffer from eating disorders more likely to try rigid diets? Or is it more likely that people on rigid diets come to have eating disorders? At this stage there just isn't enough evidence either way.

The Mayo Clinic[225] (USA) says:

"A flexible plan doesn't forbid certain foods or food groups, but instead includes a variety of foods from all the major food groups... A flexible plan allows an occasional, reasonable indulgence if you like. It should feature foods you can find in your local grocery store and that you enjoy eating. However, the plan should limit alcohol, sugary drinks and high-sugar sweets because the calories in them don't provide enough nutrients."

The second meaning of flexible dieting involves a diet that monitors the three main macronutrients: carbohydrates, fats, and proteins. The exact amounts depend on what you are trying to achieve: muscle growth, fat loss, or weight maintenance.

Emma Kinrade[226] of Glasgow Caledonian University (Scotland) sees this as an advantage over just calorie counting:

"An advantage of counting macros is that it ensures that some essential nutrients are incorporated into your diet, instead of focusing solely on calories. Counting calories takes no account of nutrients. And while it seems obvious that choosing wholesome nutritious sources of calories is better than processed, high-sugar and saturated fat foods, you could hypothetically eat seven chocolate bars (each worth 228 calories, a total of 1,596 calories) and still lose weight if your total energy expenditure is around 2,000 calories a day."

She points out that some people find counting and recording macros too difficult or time-consuming.

The other problem with this approach is that there is more to a long-term healthy diet than protein, fat and carbohydrates. It's also important to consider fibre, vitamins, minerals and phytonutrients.

111: Like What You Eat

The Mayo Clinic[227] says:

"A diet should include foods you like, that you would enjoy eating for life — not ones you can tolerate over the course of the plan. If you don't like the food on the plan, if the plan is overly restrictive or if it becomes boring, you probably won't stick to it, so long-term weight loss is unlikely."

One of the markers of a successful weight loss plan is that you could follow it for the rest of your life with a few modifications once you attain your goal weight.

The US National Institute of Diabetes And Digestive And Kidney Diseases[228] says:

"Excluding specific foods from your diet may be difficult. It may make it harder not to think about them. It's also probably unnecessary:

"You don't have to give up all your favorite foods when you're trying to lose weight. Small amounts of your favorite high-calorie foods may be part of your weight-loss plan. Just remember to keep track of the total calories you take in. To lose weight, you must burn more calories than you take in through food and beverages."

112: I'm Starving!

"I'm Starving" How often do you say this or something similar? It's very unlikely that you have ever been truly starving.

Saying "I'm starving" gives you an excuse to eat too much of the wrong type of food.

Saying "I'm a bit hungry" may be more accurate.

If you're a bit hungry, you can show restraint. If you're starving, it's understandable if you eat everything in sight.

Moderate your language, and you'll have fewer excuses to over-indulge.

113: Your To Do List

As you continue your lifelong journey toward health and fitness, remember to keep putting yourself and your needs on your to-do list! It's so easy to let the demands of family, work, friends, and other commitments take precedence in your life. For example, time for working out may get replaced by the need to chauffeur your kids to and from their scout meetings and dance classes.

Or time for preparing healthy meals may get supplanted by a work project that requires extra hours — leading to fast-food meals.

While shortchanging ourselves and our goals to meet the needs of others often seems like the right thing to do, it isn't a good long-term strategy.

Hilary Achauer[229] writes:

"I think sometimes people misunderstand what it means to "put yourself first." It doesn't mean doing what you want to do all the time. It doesn't mean ignoring the needs of others. It's all a matter of priorities and understanding the interplay between taking care of yourself and others."

She goes on to say:

"If I ignore my health, it's difficult to be there for my family, both mentally and physically."

People with children often struggle with this the most, but just think about what you are teaching your children if you are always putting other people's needs first. They will grow up without a good role model of how to take care of themselves or turn out very selfish.

If you're thinking you don't have time for yourself, check out Hack 182 Not Enough Time.

114: Carrot Or Stick

Remember the carrot-and-stick of traditional thinking? It still has relevance today. Of course, chances are you are NOT motivated by carrots, so let me put it another way: are you motivated by rewards or punishments?

Think about the past: what has motivated you to do things you didn't want to do or that were difficult? These don't have to be major goals, just tasks that you managed to complete despite yourself.

Did you plan to give yourself a reward when you completed the task? Did you think about the satisfaction you would feel when you achieved your goal? Did you think about how other people would be pleased or impressed? If these or similar approaches got you going, you are motivated by the 'carrot'. You are motivated by the positive outcomes.

Or did you think about the disappointment you would feel if you didn't succeed? Did you think about other people's disapproval? Did you deny yourself something until you completed your goal? If these or similar approaches helped, you are motivated by the 'stick'. You are motivated by negative factors.

Is it sometimes the carrot and sometimes the stick? Can you see a pattern to this? Are work goals usually motivated by the stick, and home goals by the carrot? Do you ever use both at the same time? Spend some time thinking about this, and see what patterns emerge.

Whatever they are, apply this to whatever you do to help keep you motivated to achieve your heart's desires. There isn't a wrong or right answer to this - understanding how motivation works for you will help you achieve much more in your life, including losing weight and keeping it off.

115: The Bloat

Abdominal bloating can be caused by many different factors. Gynaecological and pathological problems in the bowel should be investigated by medical professionals.

Here are just some of the other possibilities you can investigate for yourself.

Constipation can contribute to abdominal pain and bloating. If this is likely to be a problem, increase your intake of water and include more high fibre foods (see hack 104).

The website John Hopkins Medicine (USA)[230] says:

"Typically, the first line of treatment for preventing gas and bloating is changing your diet. Research has shown that a low fermentable oligosaccharides, disaccharides, monosaccharides and polyols (FODMAP) diet can reduce the symptoms of gas and IBS. A low FODMAP diet avoids fermentable, gas-producing food ingredients, such as:

- Oligosaccharides, which are found in wheat, onions, garlic, legumes and beans

- Disaccharides, such as lactose in cow's milk, yogurt and ice cream

- Monosaccharides, including fructose (a type of sugar found in fruits and honey), apples and pears

- Polyols or sugar alcohols found in foods such as apricots, nectarines, plums and cauliflower, as well as many chewing gums and candies

"In people sensitive to FODMAP-rich foods, the small intestine doesn't always fully absorb these carbohydrates, and instead passes them to the colon, where they are fermented by bacteria and produce gas. To see if some of the FODMAP foods are causing your gas and bloating you can start by cutting out FODMAP foods and then slowly bringing them back into your diet one at a time to pinpoint any foods that are causing the problems."

Stephen Norman Sullivan[231], a gastroenterologist, says:

"Physical activity seems to help bloaters and even runners and other athletes bloat less when exercising regularly."

Yet another reason to exercise regularly!

Nutritionist Anne Myers-Wright[232] says:

"There can be many causes of bloating such as eating certain foods that cause gas in the digestive tract, constipation or eating too quickly. While our go-to is often to blame a certain food or food group, if you suffer from bloating or digestive issues quite regularly and you are searching for a solution – one cause we often neglect to consider is stress!"

The brain has a direct effect on the stomach and intestines. Thinking about eating can release the stomach's digestive juices before food gets there. Your stomach or intestinal distress can be the cause or the product of anxiety, stress, or depression. That's because the brain and the gastrointestinal (GI) system are intimately connected.

Harvard Medical School (USA)[233] says:

"The gut-brain connection is no joke; it can link anxiety to stomach problems and vice versa. Have you ever had a "gut-wrenching" experience? Do certain situations make you "feel nauseous"? Have you ever felt "butterflies" in your stomach? We use these expressions for a reason. The gastrointestinal tract is sensitive to emotion. Anger, anxiety, sadness, elation — all of these feelings (and others) can trigger symptoms in the gut."

Anne Myers-Wright[234] suggests that slowing down your eating, deep belly breathing, practicing mindful eating (Hack 53) and yoga (see Hack 129) can all help.

Of course, you also need to look at what is stressing you and make any necessary changes. This may be difficult, and you may need professional help to achieve it.

116: Avocado And Belly Fat

A study led by Professor Naiman Khan[235], Illinois University (USA), looked at avocado consumption and belly/abdominal fat. The study was published in the *Journal of Nutrition*. Please note that the research was funded by the Hass Avocado Board.

The study lasted for 12 weeks. The participants were divided into two groups. One group received meals that incorporated a fresh avocado, while the other group received a meal that had nearly identical ingredients and similar calories but did not contain avocado.

Female participants who consumed an avocado a day as part of their meal had a reduction in visceral abdominal fat – the hard-to-target fat associated with higher risk – and experienced a reduction in the ratio of visceral fat to subcutaneous fat. This indicated a redistribution of fat away from the organs. However, fat distribution in males did not change, and neither males nor females had improvements in glucose tolerance. The overall weight of participants eating the avocado did not change, but the females saw a beneficial change in where the fat was located on their bodies.

Another study from the University of Illinois[236] (USA) found that eating avocado as part of your daily diet can help improve gut health. Avocados are a healthy food that is high in dietary fibre and monounsaturated fat, but the researchers did not establish how the avocados impact the microbes.

We know that gut health can affect weight loss – see Hack 62, so adding avocado may be a useful strategy for long term weight loss.

117: Backcasting

When you are thinking about your weight loss or weight maintenance goals, also spend time thinking about the steps you need to take to achieve them. Backcasting can be the best way to do this.

Think of the goal and then think of the step before you achieve the goal. Write that down. Now go backwards each time finding the step before, until you are back to today.

Now you have a detailed plan of the steps you need to take to get where you want to go. Attach dates to them, put them somewhere prominent, and tick each one off as you achieve it.

What I've just explained is when everything goes smoothly, but what if you've gone for a big goal, maybe a massive loss of weight before a big event? Backcasting will tell you if this goal is reasonable, given the time you have and your ability to eat right and exercise well. It may be the two don't fit smoothly together. Then you have to decide to change your goal, increase the time scale, double-down on your efforts or find an additional strategy.

118: Changing Your Goals

T ake a couple of moments to think of some of the important goals in your life. What are they? Do you feel motivated and energised by them?

Goals can help us get up in the morning and tackle the day with zest and enthusiasm. The extremely successful industrialist Henry Ford said:

"Obstacles are those frightful things you see when you take your eyes off your goal."

This all seems self-evidently true, but a lot of the work in this area is about goal setting in a business environment, so doesn't necessarily translate into personal goals.

A review[237] of attendees in the UK at Slimming World (a weekly commercial diet programme) concluded:

"Our analysis of a predominantly female population shows that if people with a BMI ≥ [equal to or greater than] 30 kg m^{-2} maintained attendance of a weight management group, then they were likely to achieve a clinically significant weight loss (≥10% weight loss) at 12 months irrespective of whether they set targets or not.

"Although obese and younger people were less likely to set weight-loss targets, those that did were significantly more likely to achieve a greater weight loss at 12 months than those who did not."

So, you can lose weight just through regular attendance at a weekly group, but your weight loss is likely to be greater if you also set goals.

Claire Madigan[238], senior research associate at Loughborough University (UK) writes:

"Many weight loss programmes start by asking people to set a goal. And research indeed shows that creating this "intention" actually motivates you to change your behaviour."

She goes on to say:

"Previously it was thought that goals had to be specific – for example, aiming to lose one pound a week until you've lost twenty pounds altogether. But more recent research suggests this may not be true – with data showing goal setting is effective even if the goals are vaguely defined (such as aiming to be more active, rather than aiming to run for ten minutes everyday)."

Allison Chopra[239], a fitness expert at Indiana University (USA) Chopra is a big fan of small steps and a forgiving temperament. She says:

"A goal of "eating better," is an example of a worthwhile but ambiguous goal. A more effective or specific goal might be to limit sweets to one a day for the next week or to limit cookies to the weekend...

"If a goal is not met, it should be reassessed to make sure it's reasonable and then sought after again -- after a brief break."

Faryle Nothwehr[240] and Jingzhen Yang from the University of Iowa (USA) undertook research on weight loss strategies to see if frequent revision of goals is a positive or a negative sign. They explained:

"Self-regulation theory suggests that goal setting should be an iterative process whereby the person evaluates his/her performance, and subsequently revises his/her goals or sets entirely new ones ... Thus, frequent goal setting activity might be an indicator of a stronger commitment toward behavior change ... More pessimistically, frequent goal setting could also reflect a tendency to set unrealistic goals that are not acted upon and/or require constant modification."

They found that the first possibility was correct. Frequent goal setting and goal revision mean that you're more likely to implement changes, which ultimately means you're more likely to lose weight.

The National Heart, Lung And Blood Institute[241] (USA) says:

"Shaping is a behavioral technique in which you select a series of short-term goals that get closer and closer to the ultimate goal (e.g., an initial reduction of fat intake from 40 percent of calories to 35 percent of calories, and later to 30 percent). It is based on the concept that "nothing succeeds like success." Shaping uses two important behavioral principles: (1) consecutive goals that move you ahead in small steps are the best way to reach a distant point; and (2) consecutive rewards keep the overall effort invigorated.

So, where does all this leave us? Research on goals for weight loss seems to confirm that having goals will help you lose more weight. Having smaller goals along the way is important.

But the big takeaway is that you need to keep assessing your goals. You need to review your goals to see if they are still serving you or need changing in some way. Changing your goals isn't a sign of failure. It's a sign of the dynamic and ongoing process that is involved in achieving success.

119: Feel Rather Than Achieve

People talk a lot about goals in relation to weight loss, although hack 118 shows it's a bit more complicated than it at first seems.

Some people clearly do well with a specific target weight as a goal, but it doesn't work for me. Maybe it doesn't work for you either.

Can a target weight just make you anxious? Maybe it's demotivating. Maybe you work better with feelings.

Again, it's not just some vague idea of how you want to feel at your goal. You can describe the feelings precisely.

You know how your clothes will feel. You know how you'll feel when you look in the mirror. You know how your belly will feel when you slump in front of the TV. You know how you will feel when you go to an all-you-can-eat restaurant or when someone brings your favourite cake into your home.

Get the idea? Feeling goals can be just as potent and inspiring as regular weight loss goals expressed in pounds or kilograms.

Check out Hack 179 on Visualisation too.

120: Not Just Weight Loss Goals

The British Dietetics Association[242] says:

"It's not just about your weight on the scales, losing inches from your waist helps to lower the risk of conditions like type two diabetes and high blood pressure.

"Think about goals that are not weight orientated – something else you would like to achieve such as being more active with your children or taking the stairs without getting out of breath."

Most people set weight loss goals (e.g., I want to lose 8 lbs in the next 4 weeks), but very few people set habit goals. Achieving habit goals means you are making changes that will help you keep the weight off for the rest of your life. Examples of habit goals include:

I don't always eat everything on my plate.

I rarely eat without thinking.

I don't eat while watching television.

I think about what foods I need to eat to be healthy, as well as what foods I need to eat to lose weight.

I don't put myself or other people down simply because of how much they weigh.

I don't buy high-calorie treats and gifts for other people.

121: Polyvagal Theory

Jenna Hollenstein[243], MS, RDN, CDN, describes herself as an "anti-diet dietitian". She offers the polyvagal theory as a way of understanding your relationship with food.

This theory sees three states of the autonomic nervous system. They exist like a ladder with dorsal vagal at the bottom, sympathetic in the middle, and ventral vagal at the top.

- Dorsal vagal states – shutting down or becoming immobilised when faced with a life threat. In this state you may feel sleepy and maybe you want to disappear. Eating may feel soothing and comforting even when you're not hungry.

- Sympathetic state – the flight or fight response. In this state you may feel tense, overwhelmed and trapped. May feel nauseous.

- Ventral vagal state recognises that it is belonging to a group and connecting with others that protects us. In this state you may feel content, open and receptive to others. Eating feels balanced and satisfying.

Ms Hollenstein says:

"The power of becoming familiar with your three states is recognizing them when you are there, understanding what triggers you into the dysregulated states of dorsal and sympathetic, and learning what brings you out of those dysregulated states and into the regulated ventral state. These skills can be particularly useful when dealing with the dysregulating aspects of diet culture and understanding what role food plays in nervous system regulation."

This can be a useful way of looking at what you eat. How much time today have you spent in each of these states? What causes you to go into (or stay) in the dorsal vagal state? How do you move to the ventral vagal state? Is this a helpful way to think about your relationship with food? See what insights and plans of action you can gain by looking at your eating in this way.

122: Use Therapies

Many complementary and alternative therapists can help you lose weight. Of course, some therapists will work directly on the issue of weight loss and weight maintenance. Look at Hacks 123 to 129.

Consulting a therapist about the broader picture may also be very helpful. As the American Psychological Association[244] says:

"The causes of obesity are rarely limited to genetic factors, prolonged overeating or a sedentary lifestyle. What we do and don't do often results from how we think and feel. For example, feelings of sadness, anxiety or stress often lead people to eat more than usual. Unless you act to address these emotions, however, these short-term coping strategies can lead to long-term problems ...

"Note that while treating obesity often helps decrease feelings of depression, weight loss is never successful if you remain burdened by stress and other negative feelings. You may have to work to resolve these issues first before beginning a weight-loss program."

Consulting a therapist to help with stress or negative emotions can be extremely useful. The range of therapies is huge from mainstream psychologists to alternative and complementary therapists. Even within a discipline different therapists will work slightly differently.

Ask for recommendations. Phone the therapist and have a chat, before booking an appointment. Don't be afraid to decide that a particular therapist isn't working for you but give it time. You won't necessarily see results in a couple of sessions.

But be realistic about what to expect. A good therapist is likely to help you feel better about yourself and make important changes in your life, but you are unlikely to lose as much weight as you want unless you also pay attention to what you eat.

123: Hypnotherapy

There is some evidence that hypnotherapy is beneficial for those wanting to lose wight, although most researchers add some reservations.

A study by Serpil Erşan[245] and Etem Erdal Erşan published in the *Journal Of Alternative And Complementary Medicine* says:

"This study indicates that hypnotherapy in obesity treatment leads to weight loss in obese patients and thus to considerable changes in leptin, ADP, and irisin levels [established by blood samples from participants]. Hypnotherapy is easy to apply, cheap, and effective; has no potential for side effects; and can be applied both alone and in combination with other treatments. However, to confirm its effects, further studies should be conducted on this issue."

A review of research by Nurul Afiedia Roslim[246] and colleagues published in the *Journal Of Integrative Medicine* concluded:

"... hypnotherapy has been shown to be a safe and effective adjuvant treatment for assisting weight loss. However, methodological weaknesses such as small sample sizes, high drop-out rates, therapist allegiance effects, varied techniques and duration of the hypnotherapy interventions have prevented a more concrete conclusion."

The Mayo Clinic[247] says:

"Relying on weight-loss hypnosis alone is unlikely to lead to significant weight loss, but using it as an adjunct to an overall lifestyle approach may be worth exploring for some people."

The evidence seems to suggest that hypnotherapy may be helpful for some people, but only alongside diet and lifestyle changes. The majority of hypnotherapists would not claim that you can lose weight just through hypnotherapy, but hypnotherapy can be helpful in making it easier to implement the changes you need to make in order to lose weight.

124: EFT Tapping

The Emotional Freedom Technique (EFT) involves tapping various acupuncture points using your fingers while you make various statements. It seems bizarre, but many people report that it has successfully helped them with a range of physical and psychological problems.

Peta Stapleton[248] and colleagues of Bond University, Australia compared Emotional Freedom Techniques to Cognitive Behavioural Therapy (CBT) for food cravings in adults who were overweight or obese. Data was collected at the beginning of the study, after the intervention phase (8 weeks) and at 6- and 12-months follow-up. The results were published in *Applied Psychology: Health And Well-Being*. The researchers concluded:

"Overall, EFT and CBT demonstrated comparable efficacy in reducing food cravings, one's responsiveness to food in the environment (power of food), and dietary restraint ... Results also revealed that both EFT and CBT are capable of producing treatment effects that are clinically meaningful, with reductions in food cravings, the power of food, and dietary restraint normalising to the scores of a non-clinical community sample. While reductions in BMI were not observed, the current study supports the suggestion that psychological interventions are beneficial for food cravings and both CBT and EFT could serve as vital adjunct tools in a multidisciplinary approach to managing obesity."

Dr Stapleton offers free EFT resources and paid-for programs via her website[249].

There are many anecdotal stories of people benefitting from EFT. It is a simple technique that you can learn and apply for yourself. Alternatively, you could find a therapist who practices EFT.

125: Cognitive Behavioural Therapy (CBT)

The UK NHS website[250] describes Cognitive Behavioural Therapy (CBT) like this:

"CBT is based on the concept that your thoughts, feelings, physical sensations and actions are interconnected, and that negative thoughts and feelings can trap you in a vicious cycle.

"CBT aims to help you deal with overwhelming problems in a more positive way by breaking them down into smaller parts.

"You're shown how to change these negative patterns to improve the way you feel. Unlike some other talking treatments, CBT deals with your current problems, rather than focusing on issues from your past.

"It looks for practical ways to improve your state of mind on a daily basis."

Bärbel Knäuper[251], Steven Grover and their team from McGill University (Canada) worked with nearly 200 overweight participants (both men and women) using cognitive behavioural therapy in a year-long programme. Their results suggested that cognitive behavioural therapy skills of the coaches (clinical psychology doctoral students) who delivered the program were a key factor in the treatment outcome -- as was the regular tracking of eating and physical activity using online platforms like MyFitnessPal[252] or myhealthcheckup[253].

A significant amount of weight loss was achieved. On average participants lost 10% (approximately 10kg per person) in 12 months. Group-based weight loss programs normally lead to only around 3-5% weight loss, so this is significantly higher. Crucially most participants maintained this weight loss one year after the programme ended.

A study in the UK[254] published in the *American Journal of Psychiatry*, used two versions of CBT-E [enhanced cognitive behaviour therapy]: a simple version that focused solely on the eating disorder and a second, more complex version that simultaneously addressed commonly associated problems such as low self-esteem and extreme perfectionism. Both treatments comprised twenty 50-minute outpatient appointments over twenty weeks

The researchers found that the majority of patients responded well and rapidly to the two forms of CBT-E and that the changes were sustained over the following year, the time at which relapse is most likely to occur. Approximately two-thirds of those who completed treatment made a complete and lasting response with many of the remainder showing substantial improvement.

Dr Judith Beck[255] writing in *Psychotherapy Networker* says:

"Why is it so difficult to lose weight and keep it off? By now, the "how" is no mystery: everybody knows the drill, whether you want to lose 2 pounds or 200. Just decrease your calories and get more exercise ...

"From the viewpoint of Cognitive-Behavioral Therapy (CBT), the reason isn't hard to find: knowing *what* to do and knowing *how to get yourself to do it* are entirely separate skills. When it comes to changing behavior, especially long-term, habitual patterns, getting yourself to do something different, even when you know it's good for you, depends largely on what you tell yourself: that is, on your *thinking*.

"For example, let's say you're at a dessert party and see five really delicious pastries. Will you end up eating too much? You probably will if you think, *I don't care. I don't want to deprive myself. It isn't fair that everyone else gets to eat whatever they want, and I have to settle for one small piece.* By contrast, if you say to yourself, "I'm going to pick my favorite dessert. I'll eat one small piece slowly and enjoy every bite. I know I'm going to feel so proud of myself," you stand a much better chance of not overeating."

If you decide to try CBT, and there's lots of evidence it could be helpful, look for a psychologist/psychotherapist who specialises in CBT. One that specialises in CBT for weight management would be even better.

126: Acupuncture

Kepei Zhang[256] and colleagues published a review article in *Evidence-Based Complementary And Alternative Medicine.* The research they looked at included 21 studies with 1389 participants:

"We concluded that acupuncture is an effective treatment for obesity and inferred that neuroendocrine regulation might be involved."

But the authors cautioned:

"the treatment period of obesity is rather short in many studies, varying from 3-8 weeks."

Yu-Mei Zhong[257] and colleagues did another review published in the *BMJ Postgraduate Medical Journal* and came to this conclusion:

"The review suggests that acupuncture is an effective therapy for simple obesity rather than a placebo effect. This potential benefit needs to be further evaluated by longer-term and more rigorous RCTs [randomized controlled trials]."

An article by Laila Ahmed Abou Ismail[258] and colleagues in the *Macedonian Journal Of Medical Sciences* found:

"Body acupuncture in combination with diet restriction was found to be effective for weight loss and also reduction of the inflammatory reactions. Acupuncture could be used as a synergistic treatment option for obesity control."

Note in this study they are recommending acupuncture as part of a whole programme of weight loss, not on its own.

So, like many other therapies, acupuncture appears to work well as part of an overall weight loss plan. Don't expect to go to an acupuncturist, pay them and expect that on its own to work. You have to do some work too!

127: Auricular Acupressure

Acupressure can involve the whole body or just a specific area, such as the ears (auricular acupressure) or the hands or feet. When practitioners work on a specific area, they are often affecting the whole body. So auricular acupressure is not really about the ears. There are various points on the ears that connect to various organs and systems of the whole body.

Ching-Feng Huang[259] and colleagues published a review of studies of ear acupressure in the academic journal *Medicine*.

"Pooled analysis of the 7 ... studies revealed that auricular acupressure alone, or with diet and/or exercise, was effective for weight reduction ... The study results indicate that auricular acupressure is effective for weight reduction. However, further vigorous studies that use double-blind randomized controlled design are needed to verify these findings."

Hyun Su Cha and Hyojung Park published a study in the *Journal of Korean Academy of Nursing*. This showed that auricular acupressure using vaccaria seeds was effective in decreasing body weight, abdominal circumference, body mass index, and triglyceride levels in adult women with abdominal obesity. Vaccaria seeds are traditionally used in auricular acupressure, but ceramic or metal beads are now sometimes used instead.

A study in *Advancing Digital Health And Open Science*[260] trialled a smartphone app and self-administered auricular acupressure, using six ear points. The study divided the participants into three groups:

Group 1 were taught what to do and given a booklet with information and to record their results

Group 2 had a smartphone app to remind them what to do and to log their progress

Wait group: no intervention

"The subjects in group 1 and 2 achieved better therapeutic effects in terms of body weight, body mass index (BMI), waist circumference, and hip circumference and perceived more fullness before meals than the waitlist controls."

A study by Mei-Ling Yeh[261] (National Taipei University of Nursing and Health Sciences, Taiwan) and colleagues conducted a single-blind randomised sham-controlled study on 134 participants. This meant half the participants received auricular acupressure to specific points on the ear. The other half received stimulation delivered in the same manner but at sham acupoints. All the participants received nutrition counselling by a nutritionist weekly for the 10-week study. The results were published in the *Midwest Nursing Research Society* journal. The results showed significant differences in body mass index, blood pressure, total cholesterol, triglyceride, and leptin or adiponectin over time within the group, but not between the groups. In other words acupressure was not shown to be effective.

So, there is some evidence that auricular acupressure works for weight loss, but it is not yet backed up by extensive research.

You may still want to try it to see if it is helpful for you. It is a relatively easy therapy to carry out on yourself. There are videos on YouTube, for example, which will show you how to do this for yourself.

128: Ayurveda

Ayurveda is the ancient healing system from India. If you do a web search for Ayurveda, you will see lots of listings for herbal supplements that do amazing things.

But Ayurveda is much more than this. Ayurveda classifies body types based on how much of the three Doshas (energy principals) we have within us.

Those with more Vata (air and ether) tend to be slender, and their weight fluctuates.

Pitta (fire and water) people tend to be of medium build.

Kapha (earth and water) people tend to be of a heavier build and gain weight easily.

Your body type will suggest many things. For example:

- What you need to eat

- Whether it should be mainly cooked food

- How important regular mealtimes are for you

- Whether fasting is beneficial

- Whether alcohol should not be taken

- Which herbal supplements could be beneficial

- The importance of massage, exercise and yoga

A study was published in the *Journal Of Alternative And Complementary Medicine* by Jennifer Rioux[262] and Amy Howerter of Arizona University (USA) focussing on Ayurveda and yoga for weight loss.

The study lasted for 3 months. Participants met with an Ayurvedic practitioner twice monthly (six times) and followed semi standardized dietary guidelines with individual tailoring to address relevant psychophysiological imbalances obstructing weight loss and a standardized protocol of therapeutic yoga classes three times weekly with recommended home practice of two to four additional sessions."

The researchers concluded:

"A whole-systems Ayurvedic medicine and Yoga therapy approach provides a feasible promising non-invasive low-cost alternative to traditional weight loss interventions with potential added benefits associated with sustainable holistic lifestyle modification and positive psychosocial changes."

Note that the researchers used a whole system approach rather than just prescribing Ayurvedic remedies that have traditionally been used for weight loss.

There is more research on individual compounds traditionally used within Ayurveda such as curcumin[263], berberine[264] and salacia root[265]. Some of these are showing promise, although the thrust of the research often seems to try to find the magic pharmacological compound that can be used in a magic pill for weight loss. In the long term a more wholistic approach may work better.

129: Yoga

Researchers[266] from the University of Pittsburgh (USA), Duke University Medical Center (USA) and the University of Zurich (Switzerland) studied the effect of yoga on weight loss.

50 obese or overweight adults were randomly assigned to practice either restorative hatha yoga or more vigorous vinyasa yoga, while following a 6-month behavioural weight-loss program that also included a calorie- and fat-reduced diet and a weekly group session on behavioural strategies to promote weight loss.

Participants were instructed to practice yoga 5 days per week, starting with 20 minutes per day in the first 8 weeks and progressing to 40 minutes and then 60 minutes per day. Four of the days were home-based yoga sessions, and one day involved a supervised yoga session.

People in both the restorative hatha and vinyasa yoga groups lost significant amounts of weight and improved their cardiorespiratory fitness, with no differences seen between the two styles of yoga.

Study participants saw time as a barrier to yoga participation, particularly as the length of the prescribed yoga sessions increased to 60 minutes. Although yoga was prescribed for 5 days per week, individuals tended to do it only 2 to 3 days. Even so, the majority of participants—65 percent in the hatha group and 85 percent in the vinyasa group—planned on continuing yoga after the study completed.

A study[267] published in *Evidence-Based Complementary And Alternative Medicine* studied what led yoga to work as a weight loss strategy. The researchers wanted to know if it was just that participants were exercising more or were other reasons involved.

The researchers interviewed two groups of volunteers. One group was people who had lost weight through yoga after repeatedly struggling to lose weight. The other group was those of normal weight who had lost weight unintentionally.

The researchers found that 5 themes emerged from the interviews: a shift toward healthy eating, impact of the yoga community/yoga culture, physical changes, psychological changes, and the belief that the yoga weight loss experience was different from past weight loss experiences. There were slight differences between the two groups. The researchers concluded:

"These findings imply that yoga could offer diverse behavioral, physical, and psychosocial effects that may make it a useful tool for weight loss. Role modeling and social support provided by the yoga community may contribute to weight loss, particularly for individuals struggling to lose weight."

Yoga offers many benefits, losing weight could be just one of the ones you experience.

130: In A Group Or On Your Own?

O besity researcher Dr Thomas Wadden[268], a psychology professor at the University of Pennsylvania School of Medicine (USA) says:

"Groups really provide patients a sense of universality--that they have a problem that other people share ... There is a sense of group support. People provide suggestions for each other."

Dr Katy Sutcliffe[269] of Evidence for Policy and Practice Information and Co-ordinating Centre (UK) carried out a systematic review of research on weight management programmes for people classified as overweight or obese, examining what factors contributed to successful weight loss.

She said:

"People don't have the confidence to start making changes to diet and exercise by themselves. They are more successful when they have someone to help start them off on the journey. People describe a positive sense of accountability to those individuals which helps them make changes in the short-term. Once they start to make changes they gain confidence, and begin to lose weight and feel better, this gives them the motivation to continue these measures by themselves."

A study published in the *Journal of the American Medical Association*[270] tracked 423 overweight and obese people. Half were following a programme in a group setting (Weight Watchers) and the other half followed a largely self-help approach. For this second group weight loss counselling was limited to printed material and two 20-minute sessions with a dietitian.

The study found that the commercial group's weight loss was greater than for the self-help participants. During the first year the commercial group lost on average 9.5 lbs. The self-help group lost on average 3 lbs.

In the second year the commercial group's participants held onto a 6.4-pound loss overall and the self-help group members returned to their pre-study weight.

Researchers from Drexel University[271] (USA) studied 87 adult participants in a 12-month weight loss programme. For the entire study participants were asked to complete three self-monitoring activities daily – wear a Fitbit fitness tracker, weigh themselves on a wireless scale and log their food intake in a smartphone app.

For the first three months of the study all participants started with a weekly group session to learn behavioural skills. After the third month, the group sessions ended. From that point through the end of the study (9 months) – known as the maintenance phase – each participant received just one weekly text message and one monthly phone call with their coach.

During the maintenance phase, half the participants worked with a coach who had access to their self-monitoring data. The coach addressed the data during the phone calls and text messages. The coaches for the other half of the participants could not see the data from the Fitbit, wireless scale or digital food record.

The researchers concluded that, although the study was small, the pattern suggests that when coaches had access to data, it helped participants keep off their weight.

In this study the person who saw the data was a professional, so we do not know if it would also apply if the person who saw the data was a friend or relative. You may not have a chance to work with a professional, so you could try this and see if it works using a supportive friend or colleague.

The US National Weight Control Registry[272] is a research study that seeks to gather information from people who have successfully lost weight and kept it off. In order to participate people need to meet all these criteria:

18 years or over

Lost at least 30 pounds, and

Maintained a weight loss of at least 30 pounds for one year or more

The participants are sent questionnaires from time to time, which ask about their success at losing weight, current weight maintenance strategies and other health-related behaviours. These are completed online.

The website says they have over 10,000 members in the registry that was established in 1994 by scientific researchers. Not all of them would respond to a particular questionnaire. They have found:

"45% of registry participants lost the weight on their own and the other 55% lost weight with the help of some type of program."

So though more people achieved success using a programme, lots of people did it on their own. This is much higher than the other research suggests. This may be that people who like to do things on their own are more likely to sign up to the Registry.

In general, being part of a group seems to be helpful for a lot of people, but if you're someone who generally likes to go it alone, don't feel you have to join a group to succeed.

131: Social Support

We know that many people benefit from losing weight in a group or with a coach, but what about with more general support from family and friends?

A study from the University of Illinois[273] (USA) led by Catherine J. Metzgar conducted focus groups with 23 women about a year and a half after they completed a weight-loss program to determine which factors helped or hindered dieters' success.

All the women who participated had lost a significant amount of weight on the programme, but many were unsuccessful at maintaining it after the programme ended.

A major obstacle for some of these dieters was a lack of social support from significant people in their lives. Rather than encouraging the dieters' efforts to get healthier, some friends and family members responded negatively. They intentionally or unintentionally sabotaged progress by making unhelpful comments or tempting them with high-calorie foods.

The women who maintained their weight loss indicated that a high level of social support from many sectors was critical in their success.

Dr Metzgar commented:

"What this study shows is that if you can find that one friend who has the same goals or can just hold you accountable, it is really helpful."

Assistant professor Amy McQueen[274] (Washington University In St Louis, USA) says:

"Not everyone needs social support to change every habit, but the ones that are more social in nature (like going out to eat with others) may require some negotiation and invitations for support. Family members who do not support healthy-eating intentions or tobacco-cessation attempts will make it much harder for the person trying to make a change to succeed. Co-workers can be helpful by not always bringing in cookies and cakes to the office and by suggesting walking or stretching breaks or meetings."

And the extra twist to this is that researchers[275] from Ohio State University (USA) have found that being willing to give social support to your spouse, friends and family may be just as important as receiving assistance in terms of your health. There is a positive benefit for the person offering the support as well as the one receiving the support.

132: Spouses

Sadly, spouses and partners aren't always helpful, but weight loss can be more successful if they join you in your effort.

Lotte Verweij[276], Amsterdam University of Applied Sciences (Netherlands) looked at heart attack survivors engaging with a programme that focussed on weight reduction, increasing physical activity, and stopping smoking. She said:

"Our study shows that when spouses join the effort to change habits, patients have a better chance of becoming healthier - particularly when it comes to losing weight."

Compared to those without a partner, patients with a participating partner were more than twice as likely to improve in at least one of the three areas (weight loss, exercise, smoking cessation) within a year.

This is a big difference. Is it time to have a chat with your spouse or partner? Maybe show them the research.

133: 12 Step Programmes

Everyone's heard of the 12 step programme for alcoholics, better known as Alcoholics Anonymous. This approach can also be used for those who want to gain control of their eating.

The website 12step.com[277] says:

"At the heart of any 12 step program is a realization that one's life has spiraled out of control. Help is needed. Those who struggle with their weight can feel just as helpless as others and the structure of a 12 step program, along with the support provided in a group, can mean the difference between success and continued failure."

12 Step programs for weight loss are run by various organisations including Overeaters Anonymous and Food Addicts Anonymous (now, Food Addicts in Recovery Anonymous[278]).

The 12 steps as outlined by Overeaters Anonymous[279] are:

1. We admitted we were powerless over food — that our lives had become unmanageable.

2. Came to believe that a Power greater than ourselves could restore us to sanity.

3. Made a decision to turn our will and our lives over to the care of God as we understood Him.

4. Made a searching and fearless moral inventory of ourselves.

5. Admitted to God, to ourselves and to another human being the exact nature of our wrongs.

6. Were entirely ready to have God remove all these defects of character.

7. Humbly asked Him to remove our shortcomings.

8. Made a list of all persons we had harmed and became willing to make amends to them all.

9. Made direct amends to such people wherever possible, except when to do so would injure them or others.

10. Continued to take personal inventory and when we were wrong, promptly admitted it.

11. Sought through prayer and meditation to improve our conscious contact with God as we understood Him, praying only for knowledge of His will for us and the power to carry that out.

12. Having had a spiritual awakening as the result of these Steps, we tried to carry this message to compulsive overeaters and to practice these principles in all our affairs.

Some people struggle with the spiritual nature of some of the steps, but the organisation says it has agnostics and atheists who are members.

The Wikipedia entry[280] on Overeaters Anonymous (retrieved January 2022) says:

"The average weight loss of participants in OA has been found to be 21.8 pounds (9.9 kg). Survey results show that 90 percent of OA has responded that they have improved "somewhat, much, or very much" in their emotional, spiritual, career and social lives. OA's emphasis on group commitment and psychological and spiritual development provided a framework for developing positive, adaptive and self-nurturing treatment opportunities."

And the Wikipedia entry[281] for Food Addicts in Recovery Anonymous says

"A self-published survey of FA membership in 2011 showed 80% of members had lost 25 lbs. or more, and of those, 50% were at their goal weight. At that time, 33% of FA members had over 13 months of recovery from food addiction, and 22% had between 3 and 30 years with no return to food addiction."

The evidence seems to be clear that 12-step programmes run by various organisations work well for some people. Are you one of the people it would work well for?

134: Weighing Yourself Every Day

A study by Carly R. Pacanowski[282] and David A. Levitsky in the *Journal of Obesity* looked at daily self-weighing. The researchers concluded:

"Self-weighing and visual feedback may be a useful strategy combined with other techniques to promote healthful weight loss."

Carol Shieh[283] and colleagues agree:

"Self-weighing is likely to improve weight outcomes, particularly when performed daily or weekly, without causing untoward adverse effects."

Jeffrey J VanWormer[284] and colleagues ran a six-month project that included self-weighing:

"Self-weighing may be a strategy to enhance behavioral weight-loss programs. Weekly self-weighing seems to be a reasonable, evidence-supported recommendation for successful weight loss."

Claire D. Madigan[285] and colleagues looked at randomised control trial research in this area and concluded:

"There is a lack of evidence of whether advising self-weighing without other intervention components is effective. Adding self-weighing to a behavioural weight loss programme may improve weight loss. Behavioural weight loss programmes that include self-weighing are more effective than minimal interventions. Accountability may improve the effectiveness of interventions that include self-weighing."

They also found "There was no significant difference in the interventions with weekly or daily weighing."

The researchers are suggesting it is not enough on its own. Adding in accountability can make it more effective. This means sharing your results with someone else each time you do it.

But another study by researchers in Finland[286] was more positive about the benefits of self-weighing:

"Frequent self-weighing was associated with favorable weight loss outcomes also in an uncontrolled, free-living setting, regardless of specific weight loss interventions. The beneficial associations of regular self-weighing were more pronounced for overweight or obese individuals."

Overall most researchers seem to be saying that self-weighing is beneficial when used as part of an overall strategy.

The research doesn't seem to come down in favour of daily or weekly weighing. This may be something you need to try for yourself to find out which works better for you.

The US National Heart, Lung & Blood Institute[287] says:

When weighing yourself and keeping a weight graph or table, however, remember that one day's diet and exercise patterns won't have a measurable effect on your weight the next day. Today's weight is not a true measure of how well you followed your program yesterday, because your body's water weight will change from day to day, and water changes are often the result of things that have nothing to do with your weight-management efforts.

If you're weighing every day, you need to be looking at the trend. Is your weight going up over time or is it staying roughly the same or decreasing? Getting depressed or angry because you are a tiny bit heavier today than you were yesterday is neither useful nor helpful.

135: Meal Replacements

An article[288] published in the academic journal *Obesity Reviews* looked at research into the effectiveness of meal replacements. They looked at research where at least one meal per day was replaced, but also included at least one meal comprising conventional foods.

"The key finding of this review is that participants assigned to a MR [meal replacement] diet compared with a diet only approach (akin to a self-directed weight loss attempt) lose an additional 1.44 kg at 1 year, and this difference appears to be maintained up to 4 years."

Research[289] published in the *Journal of Obesity* aimed to evaluate the impact of meal replacement in individuals (from a Chinese population) who were overweight or obese. The control group continued as normal, whereas the intervention group had a dinner replacement of 388 kcal for 12 weeks. The researchers concluded:

"A 12-week meal replacement with mild caloric restriction study conducted in a group of Chinese participants with overweight and obesity showed significant reduction or improvement in 14 body composition parameters as well as 3 out of 7 metabolic parameters assessed."

They go on to say:

"... the overall loss of 4.3% body weight coincides with clinically significant improvements in blood pressure (males only) and glucose (males and females) levels."

Michelle Kulovitzand[290] and Len Kravitz of the University of New Mexico (USA) caution:

"If utilizing one meal replacement per day a person can continue indefinitely, as long as he/she monitors intake at other meals to maintain a well-balanced diet. If the plan is to utilize two or more meal replacements per day it is recommended that the client seek the advice of a clinical weight loss specialist."

Nerys Astbury[291], senior researcher in diet and obesity at the University of Oxford (UK) says:

"Our review showed that risk factors for disease including HbA1c, a blood marker used to diagnose type 2 diabetes, improved more in people using meal replacement than in those using other types of weight loss programme.

"If you're considering losing weight, our latest evidence suggests that replacement diets can be a sound option."

I've written all this with gritted teeth. I've always felt like meal replacements are a poor choice. Much better to eat a healthy diet and make behavioural changes. But I'm committed to sharing with you what the evidence says. The evidence doesn't agree with my views!

Meal replacements seem to be particularly effective when people struggle with portion control. They are definitely an option at least for one meal a day.

136: Alcohol And Calories

R esearch[292] from Alcohol Change UK has shown that the general population has a relatively poor awareness of the number of calories in their drinks. A survey of over 2,000 UK adults in 2014 showed that over 80% of people did not know or underestimated the number of calories in a large glass of wine, and over 60% of people did not know or underestimated the number of calories in a pint of lager

Alcohol Change UK[293] give these figures:

- Standard glass of wine(175ml) is around 158 calories

- Large glass of wine (250 ml) is around 225 calories

- Beer, lager, cider (1Pint or 568ml) is around 222 calories

- Spirits (neat, 25 ml) is around 50 calories.

James Brown[294], Associate Professor in Biology and Biomedical Science, Aston University (UK), writes in *The Conversation*:

"Two glasses of wine might add more sugar to your diet than eating a doughnut"

You can see that spirits (such as whisky, gin and vodka) have fewer calories, but there are other health reasons to keep your consumption of spirits low.

In a study some years ago they found that 43% of people in a survey who kept track of calories did not include calories from alcohol as part of this! The term "beer belly" did not come about for no reason.

You're only fooling yourself if you do this.

The Heart Research Institute UK[295] says:

"Too much alcohol can sap your energy, cause an intake of excess kilojoules (calories), deplete important energy-releasing B vitamins, and cause headaches and an inability to concentrate. Following the rule of twos is a great guide to alcohol consumption if you like to enjoy a drink."

They recommend the rule of twos:

"Two a day is plenty. Have two 'miss a drink' days a week. Two times two is a treat, and two treats a week is too many."

If you find it difficult to moderate your alcohol intake, consider Hack 08 on variety. Reduce the variety of alcohol you have available at home.

Of course, complete abstinence from alcohol is the only way forward for some people.

137: Alcohol And Appetite

The NI Direct Government Services website[296] (Northern Ireland) says:

"Drinking a small amount of alcohol stimulates your appetite because it increases the flow of stomach juices."

This can mean that you feel hungrier than you actually are. If you're wanting to control your food intake, you are making it harder for yourself if you drink even a small amount of alcohol.

If you drink more alcohol, your inhibitory controls are likely to be affected. In other words, drinking alcohol can make it hard for you to think clearly and make good decisions. Your desire to eat well can easily disappear as you drink more. You knew that didn't you?

The American Addictions Centers' website[297] describes it like this:

"Alcohol also decreases some of the activity of the prefrontal cortex. This part of the brain is what helps you to think clearly and rationally, and it is involved in your decision making abilities. When you drink, alcohol makes it harder for the prefrontal cortex to work as it should, disrupting decision-making and rational thought. In this way, alcohol prompts you to act without thinking about your actions."

Is it easier for you to refuse all alcohol at social events?

If this won't work for you, what can you do to moderate the effects of alcohol? Alternating an alcoholic drink with a glass of water or a non-alcoholic drink works for some people.

138: Fat Shaming & Fat Talk

Fat shaming doesn't help people lose weight. That's very clear from the research in this area. In fact, it may well do the opposite – stop them losing weight or even mean they put weight on.

Studies show that exposure to weight bias often results in physiological and behavioural changes linked to poor metabolic health and increased weight gain.

Assistant professor Angela Alberga[298] says:

"You actually experience a form of stress [when you are fat shamed] ... Cortisol spikes, self-control drops and the risk of binge eating increases."

She goes on to say:

"It's a really complex relationship that goes beyond energy-in-energy-out ... It's estimated that two in five Americans with a higher than "normal" BMI have internalized weight bias."

Internalised weight bias means you think of yourself negatively in relation to your weight. You maybe think you are weak-willed, stupid, disgusting or shameful. Maybe you think you are ugly or unattractive.

The US National Eating Disorders Association[299] offers 10 tips To Positive Body Image on their website:

1. Appreciate all that your body can do.

2. Keep a top-ten list of things you like about yourself—things that aren't related to how much you weigh or what you look like.

3. Remind yourself that "true beauty" is not simply skin-deep.

4. Look at yourself as a whole person. When you see yourself in a mirror or in your mind, choose not to focus on specific body parts.

5. Surround yourself with positive people.

6. Shut down those voices in your head that tell you your body is not "right" or that you are a "bad" person. [See also hack 143 Self-Talk]

7. Wear clothes that are comfortable and that make you feel good about your body.

8. Become a critical viewer of social and media messages.

9. Do something nice for yourself — something that lets your body know you appreciate it [See Hack 170 on 25 Ways To Reward Yourself].

10. Use the time and energy that you might have spent worrying about food, calories, and your weight to do something to help others.

Some of these suggestions may feel difficult but start with the easiest one and see if you can get better at that.

In an interesting study by Viren Swami, Professor of Social Psychology, Anglia Ruskin University (UK) published in the journal *Body Image*[300] almost 400 adults in the US completed a questionnaire about the amount of time they spent in nature in everyday life and activities. They also completed measures of self-esteem and "body appreciation".

Body appreciation is about the extent to which people hold favourable opinions about their bodies, accept and respect their bodies, and reject unrealistic beauty standards. He found that both women and men who reported greater exposure to nature also reported more positive body appreciation.

There are a lot of reasons to spend more time in nature. Feeling more positive about your body is just one of them.

And, of course, it's not just thoughts about yourself. Also pay attention to conversations you have with other people. Do you talk to close friends in a way that fat shames you both? Do you look at other people and judge them by their weight?

Changing these negative thoughts and behaviour doesn't happen overnight. But not dealing with it will make it more difficult for you to lose weight and keep it off. It will also make it more difficult if you are supporting someone else to become a healthy weight.

139: Stronger And Thinner

Professor Kathleen Martin Ginis[301] of the University of British Columbia (Canada) says:

"Women, in general, have a tendency to feel negatively about their bodies. This is a concern because poor body image can have harmful implications for a woman's psychological and physical health including increased risk for low self-esteem, depression and for eating disorders."

Martin Ginis, along with her graduate student Lauren Salci, compared the body image and physical perceptions of women who completed 30 minutes of moderate aerobic exercise with those who sat and read. Women in the exercise group had significant improvements in their body image compared to those who didn't exercise.

This positive effect lasted at least 20 minutes post-exercise. The research team further established that this effect was not due to a change in the women's mood, rather it was linked to perceiving themselves as stronger and thinner.

"We all have those days when we don't feel great about our bodies," says Martin Ginis. "This study and our previous research shows one way to feel better, is to get going and exercise. The effects can be immediate."

You may be thinking that an effect that lasts 20 minutes is not worth working out for! But you can hopefully build on that more positive feeling for the rest of your day.

140: Take Part In A Trial

S cientists all round the world are looking for people to take part in research on obesity. You could be a participant in one of these trials and may lose weight. Of course, there's no guarantee of this. You could end up in the control group or the intervention itself may not work.

The easiest way to find a trial local to you seems to be using the website clinicaltrials.g ov[302]. This lists trials in many different countries. It is maintained by the US government, so all the trials will have to follow ethical standards.

At the time of writing (2022), the website search function is not very user-friendly. They have a version in beta, which is much easier to use: beta.clinicaltrials.gov[303] Being in beta means it has some imperfections, but if you struggle with the main site, do try the beta site.

Of course, there may not be a trial near you, but it is worth doing the search to find out.

Alternatively, you could contact your local university or similar institution and find out if they do research on obesity and need volunteers.

Be careful about participating in a trial by a random company you find on the internet. You want to participate in a trial that will protect your health and wellbeing.

141: Parents

Some people attribute their problems with food and their weight to their parents.

Did your parents show you love through food?

Were you made to eat up all the food on your plate?

Was nice food withheld when you were naughty?

Did you see your parents using excessive alcohol to numb their feelings?

These and other actions of your parents can add to the difficulty of gaining a healthy weight, but they are not insurmountable.

Blaming our parents is easy. It gives us permission to stay exactly the way we are. But it's hard, because it means we stay where we are – in our pain, anger and/or dysfunctional behaviour.

Do you still behave in the same way around food, even though you're a grown-up and allowed so many other things to change? Think of all the things that have changed in your life since you were a child. Maybe write them down.

How did you change those things? Can you use the same strategies to make changes around your relationship with food?

Of course, if you're blaming your parents for how you are, you have to let them blame their parents for how they are. It's not logical to say they're to blame for how you are and also for how they are.

Maybe the messages weren't that direct. Maybe your parents undermined your confidence, so that you feel even now that things are difficult for you, that change is scary and that it's better not to be noticed.

What did your parents say that started with:

You'll never ...

You'll always ...

Men should/can't …

Women should/can't …

When you've worked out a few of the messages, take just one. Think about how you can change the message. Here are some examples:

"You'll never be any good."

List all the things you are good at. Ask friends and supportive loved ones for ideas if you can't think of many yourself. Put them on notes and stick them round the house so you can see them or write them in a book and read it first thing in the morning or last thing at night.

"You'll always be fat. It runs in the family."

Look at the research about how effective exercise and a healthy diet is in maintaining a good shape. Ask your slim friends if any of them have fat parents. Get yourself a personal trainer. Read this book from cover to cover!

J.K. Rowling has said:

"There is an expiry date on blaming your parents for steering you in the wrong direction."

Psychologist Dr Joshua Coleman[304] and colleagues have written a blog post called "The Cost of Blaming Parents":

"One of the biggest dangers of carrying chronic feelings of anger toward a parent lies not simply in what it does to the relationship between us and our parents, but how it might affect our relationships with an intimate partner or our children."

It also distorts your relationship with yourself.

I'm not saying it's easy. You have to keep working at it. Take one small part of the messages and focus on that. It may be hard work, but isn't it a better alternative than locking yourself into a future that's determined by the past? How long have you been an adult? How long were you a child? How many more years have you got to live? Live them as a strong adult not a hurt child.

You may be able to do this on your own, or you may need to find a therapist to help you.

142: Punitive Parent

For some people early childhood experiences run deep. Dysfunctional eating patterns and habits in overweight and obese adults can be triggered by early life experiences. These may become deeply rooted and difficult to change.

Professor Barbara Basile[305] of the School of Cognitive Psychotherapy (Italy) explains the result of her study:

""Our findings highlight the role of the Insufficient Self-Control schema among overweight and obese individuals, which manifests as difficulties in tolerating distress and restraining impulses. We also documented that overeating and bingeing behaviors serve as self-soothing strategies that help individuals to cut off their feelings and quiet their internalized 'Punitive Parent'."

She says that to help people with these deep-rooted challenges work needs to be done to:

- Address and satisfy the frustrated core emotional needs, embedded in the vulnerable child mode, in a safe therapeutic relationship.

- De-potentiate the punitive parental mode and its destructive messages.

- Reduce dysfunctional coping mechanisms.

- Expand the healthy adult mode.

These sorts of changes may not be amenable to simple hacks or short-term changes, but may need an ongoing, long-term relationship with a therapist specialising in this area.

143: Negative Self-Talk

Many of us experience this voice in our head, telling us we are not good enough or we can't do this, or no one will ever like us.

If you're trying to gain mastery over what you eat, it can be really hard if you have a voice in your head telling you that you will not succeed.

You may accept that self-talk, at least in part, determines our reality. You know that it doesn't make sense to say to yourself "I can't do this" just before you try! But you may find it impossible to stop that voice.

Much of the advice about dealing with negative self-talk comes down to suppressing it, being critical of yourself, being the jailer of your thoughts.

You're constantly waiting, listening: "Oh, there I go again. I've got to stop this." That can be successful to some extent, but how can you feel positive and relaxed about yourself while you use this strategy?

So, you need a different approach.

A deceptively simple strategy comes from T Harv Eker[306], who's an online coach for personal and business development. He suggests that when you catch yourself doing negative self-talk, you say to yourself "four magic words". The magic words are:

Thank you for sharing.

Four very simple words. He says it is important to do it kindly. Remember, you're speaking to your bodyguard, your over-worrying mother, the small child who was bullied or slapped down. The voice is doing its best to keep you safe, even though situations may have changed.

Be gentle. Don't be aggressive or critical of what you're thinking. Just realise that this part of you is doing its best to protect you in a dangerous world. Just because it's doing its best, it doesn't mean it's telling you the truth. Sometimes these thoughts might have been very useful at a particular time in your life, but it doesn't mean they are now. In fact, they're very unlikely to be useful now, because your circumstances have changed from when that self-talk first started, which is often when you were a small child.

You are in a much more powerful place than when you were a small child. So, the negative self-talk that was appropriate, that kept you safe, kept you out of danger as a small child may no longer be appropriate.

But remember, you're not trying to suppress it. You're not getting angry. You are simply saying, "Thank you for sharing."

It's simple, but it can be highly effective. You can acknowledge the voice and move on.

144: Your Power

Are you giving away your power?

When you eat in a restaurant, buy a ready meal, buy chocolate or an ice cream, do you let the producer decide what is the amount you should eat by finishing whatever the portion size happens to be?

Take back your power and decide for yourself when you've had enough.

Do store owners decide your impulse buys by putting high calorie food next to the checkout?

Take back your power and choose for yourself what you buy.

145: Interoception

M elissa Barker [307] and Rebecca Brewer of Royal Holloway University of London (UK) describe interoception like this:

"Interoception includes perceiving various internal sensations from the body. It means noticing things like how quickly your heart is beating, how heavily you are breathing, how hot or cold you are, and whether you are feeling hungry or full. It can occur without us even knowing it, for example, when our body regulates our blood sugar levels. Or it can be very noticeable, such as our heart thumping when we give a presentation.

"It makes sense that these difficulties would be linked to eating disorders. If you struggle to notice when you are hungry, you may under-eat. And if you struggle to notice when you are full, you may binge eat."

The researchers go on to say that at the moment it is unclear which comes first – interoception, emotional problems or eating disorders.

You may be wondering what use this information is to you! Interoception is yet another way of looking at what is going on in your body. How good are you at noticing when your heart rate is up or your palms are sweaty? What happens in your body when your blood sugar drops? If you're really hungry, what happens in your body?

Spending some time interrogating your body in this way may help you notice the signals that your body is giving you to say it is full and doesn't need any more food. Could you get better at interoception if you tried?

146: Clearing Your Plate

Y ou may have been taught to clear your plate as a child. That early childhood messaging can seem difficult to break. It's an important one to break. Not surprisingly, research confirms that "the tendency to clear one's plate when eating is associated with increased body weight and may constitute a risk factor for weight gain".

This comment comes from a study of 993 people in the US, published in the research journal *Obesity*[308]. Participants were asked about their tendency to clear their plate and always finish a meal. Their BMIs were measured and the study concluded that "plate clearing was significantly positively associated with BMI".

This is something that may need work on over time. Don't get discouraged. It can be hard to change those habits learned as a child, particularly ones linked to parental approval. But it can be done.

147: Food & Love

"But I made these treats especially for you!" or some variation of that can seem like a situation where you have to eat whatever is on offer and have seconds (and thirds?) too in order not to upset the person who's made this especially for you.

If possible, have a discussion with the person outside of the situation. So, if your mum always tries to feed you up when you visit, try to talk about it at some other time.

It's important to recognise that the person doing this is trying to show you love, so you need to start by recognising that. Also, you need to validate the person's skills too. So, saying things like this may help:

"I know you really love/like me and want me to be happy."

"You are such a great baker."

Put the onus for the problem on yourself:

"The trouble is once I start eating cake, I just can't stop. Then I feel sick/sad/spotty. I know you want me to be happy, so please can you not make me cake. I know you love me even when you don't bake me a cake."

But what to do in the moment if you're faced with the cake. Dr. Susan Albers[309] says that you can simply say "no thanks":

"The key is *how* you say it. Say it with force and conviction... Food is a connector. It can be an expression of love. When someone uses food to strengthen the bond, try other ways to let them know you care. Verbal 'I love yous!' and compliments can reaffirm these connections without calories."

Don't just assume that you must accept food that's given with love. Spend some time to see if you can find a way that minimises the hurt for the person giving food as love. Remember they are probably doing the best they can.

148: Who Are You Kidding?

D o you convince yourself that you need to buy high calorie foods, so your children or partner won't feel deprived? Then you somehow find yourself eating them?

Do the ones you love need or want these high calorie foods? Are you really buying for them or is it an excuse to buy for yourself?

Be honest with yourself.

149: Forced To Be Bad

Fangyuan Chen and Jaideep Sengupta[310] from Hong Kong University of Science and Technology looked at decisions around desserts and other indulgent food. They say:

"Imagine you're dining out with a friend who insists on sharing some chocolate cake for dessert. Since the decision has already been made for you, you gladly join in without feeling any regret.

"Most of us don't like being forced to do things. The freedom to make our own decisions generally energizes us and increases our sense of well-being. However, when it comes to purchasing and consuming products normally associated with feelings of guilt, reducing someone's sense of free choice could ultimately boost their overall well-being,"

The researchers say:

"In an effort to avoid punishment, children will say someone else 'made them' break the rules. As it turns out, this evasion of responsibility also works surprisingly well for adults and may carry substantial benefits for consumers."

The authors talk about benefits, but the benefits are often only when you take a short-term view. Long term if you keep consuming that cake you will put on weight.

Being aware of how this dynamic works can help you guard against it.

150: Do Your Own Shopping

Researcher Juliano Laran[311] of the University of Miami (USA) found that consumers exert more self-control when they make choices for themselves. They purchase less healthy foods when buying for others. In his research participants were faced with healthy and indulgent food. He found:

"When making choices for themselves, participants chose a balance of healthy and indulgent food items," Laran writes. "When making choices for others, however, participants chose mostly indulgent food items."

He goes on to say:

"One of the reasons the population gets more and more obese is that a lot of the food we consume is chosen by other people, like friends throwing a party or parents buying for their children... Taking responsibility for their own choices instead of letting others choose could help consumers fight against obesity and lead a healthier lifestyle."

This is an interesting piece of research – if you would choose healthy food for yourself, why are you assuming other people want unhealthy food?

Do you feel distressed when someone buys you something high-calorie? Even if you do, you probably don't say anything, because you won't want to hurt the other person's feelings. Maybe you're really enthusiastic conveying to them that they've done the right thing. Maybe next time you buy for someone else, take a moment to consider is that really what they would want.

151: Pay With Cash

It may be a while since you've used cash, but it could be a help in your desire to eat more healthily.

Studies have shown that you are likely to spend more on impulsive buys when you are making a cashless purchase.

Joowon Park[312] and colleagues from the University of Chicago (USA) found:

"when participants in our studies considered making cash payments, the negative arousal caused by the pain of paying directed their attention to the health risk, which reduced their purchase likelihood and their willingness to pay. However, when the participants considered making cashless payments, the absence of the negative arousal reduced their attention to the health risks, which increased their purchase likelihood and their willingness to pay."

So, here's a simple hack. Carry some cash and pay using cash whenever possible for impulsive buys.

152: Distractions

Professor Martin Yeomans[313] from the School of Psychology at the University of Sussex (UK) found in his research that

"... if you're eating or drinking while your attention is distracted by a highly engaging task, you're less likely to be able to tell how full you feel. You're more likely to keep snacking than if you'd been eating while doing something less engaging.

"This is important for anyone wanting to stay a healthy weight: if you're a habitual TV-watching snacker -- watching, say, an engaging thriller or mystery, or a film with a lot of audio or visual effects -- you're not likely to notice when you feel full.

"Video-gamers and crossword solvers should also take note!"

Eric Robinson and colleagues reviewed various studies and published their findings in the American Journal Of Clinical Nutrition[314]. They found:

"Evidence indicates that attentive eating is likely to influence food intake and incorporation of attentive-eating principles into interventions may aid weight loss and maintenance without the need for conscious calorie counting."

If you pay attention while you're eating, you're more likely to recognise when you've had enough. You are also likely to get more pleasure out of it too.

See also Hack 54 Mindfully Eating A Raisin.

153: Screen Time

When eating or snacking in front of the TV, put the amount that you plan to eat into a bowl or container instead of eating straight from the package. It's easy to overeat when your attention is focused on something else. Better still, don't eat while you watch TV.

Professor Stuart Biddle[315] of Loughborough University (UK) says:

"Not only are television viewers exposed to numerous advertisements that can influence the type of food they desire and consume, but television can also act as a distraction, resulting in a lack of awareness of actual food consumption or overlooking food cues that may lead to overconsumption.

"For some people, a substantial proportion of their daily energy intake is consumed whilst watching TV."

The World Cancer Research Fund International[316] says:

"When using screens, we are typically inactive and use up little energy. This displaces time that could be spent being more physically active. Being inactive can disrupt our normal appetite signalling and lead to passively eating more than is needed. Screen time can also increase exposure to marketing of foods and drinks that promote weight gain."

The Fund also says:

"Overweight and obesity are causally linked to 12 cancers[317], so the drivers of weight gain, overweight and obesity are also indirectly the drivers of cancer risk."

As well as weight gain, television watching can hamper weight maintenance when you've lost that excess weight. Douglas A Raynor[318] and colleagues found:

"Individuals who are successful at maintaining weight loss over the long term are likely to spend a relatively minimal amount of time watching TV."

You may not watch a lot of television, but any sort of screen watching is likely to reduce your awareness of what you are eating if you eat at the same time. Screen time usually means a time of limited physical activity too.

If you find yourself, glued to your mobile phone, consider buying a basic phone that only offers phone calls and texts and use this some of the time.

154: Perseverance

Getting control of your weight and how you feel about your body is not down to any quick fixes. It takes time and perseverance.

Ian Hamilton[319] (Associate Professor, Addiction and Mental Health, University of York, UK) and Sally Marlow (Addictions Researcher, King's College London, UK) are talking about drug addiction, but has relevance for weight loss too:

"Perseverance underpins most stories of successful change, and it can take anywhere from six to 30 attempts to quit for those dependent on drugs to become abstinent. While these numbers might seem off putting, it's important to be realistic about the need to persevere. Incremental change is known to be superior to overly ambitious targets – appealing as they might be."

They go on to say:

"Having a lapse shouldn't be viewed as a failure or used as an excuse to give up. It can be tempting to view change in a binary way - success or failure. Instead, view a lapse as an opportunity to gain insight, reflecting as honestly as possible on why the lapse happened and how this could be avoided or counteracted on the next attempt at change."

Life coach Michael Pollock[320] says:

"According to decades of research, there are two fundamental belief systems, also known as "mindsets," that determine how people respond to struggle, setbacks and failure when pursuing their goals. In one mindset, you're likely to get discouraged and give up on your goal. In the other, you tend to embrace the struggle, learn from the setbacks and keep moving forward – you persevere."

Which mindset do you have? If you want to gain control, you need to cultivate the perseverance mindset. Do you need to spend less time looking for magic solutions and more time changing your mindset? I love this quote from John D Rockefeller:

"I do not think that there is any other quality so essential to success of any kind as the quality of perseverance. It overcomes almost everything, even nature."

155: Implementation Intentions

"I mplementation intentions" are what psychologists call "if .. then" plans.

Examples include:

If Mary insists on giving me a box of chocolates, I'll thank her and give it secretly to a foodbank.

If I'm within 200 steps of my goal for the day, I'll walk round the house till I reach it.

If I have a really bad day with eating, I'll focus on eating extra fibre the next day.

Get the idea?

The concept of implementation intentions was introduced in 1999 by psychologist Peter Gollwitzer. Studies conducted by Gollwitzer in 1997 and earlier show that the use of implementation intentions can result in an increased probability of successfully reaching your goal.

Brian Harman[321] (De Montfort University, UK) and Professor Janine Bosak (Dublin City University, Ireland) write on The Conversation website:

" ... [a] meta-analysis of 94 studies informs us that "implementation intentions" are also highly effective. These personalised "if x then y" rules can counter the automatic activation of habits. For example, if I feel like eating chocolate, I will drink a glass of water.

"Implementation intentions with multiple options are very effective since they provide the flexibility to adapt to situations. For example, "if I feel like eating chocolate I will (a) drink a glass of water, (b) eat some fruit; or (c) go for a walk".

"But negatively framed implementation intentions ("when I feel like eating chocolate, I will not eat chocolate") can be counterproductive since people have to suppress a thought ("don't eat chocolate")." [See Hack 03]

Get the idea? Can you set yourself some "If ... then" scenarios to help you on your weight management journey?

156: Vice Foods

What do you call those "naughty but nice" treats you have occasionally? Some researchers call them "vice food".

Researchers[322] at Cornell University (USA) asked a group of undergraduates to rate 100 food categories according to impulsiveness. The researchers found not surprisingly that impulsiveness was highly associated with unhealthy foods.

"Beans, barley, rice, baby food, vegetables, milk, and meat were some of the less impulsive categories, and ice cream, candies, cookies, gum, donuts, potato chips, and pudding were some of the more impulsive product categories"

They then created a vice index – a combination of impulsiveness and unhealthiness. You probably already have a good idea of which had the highest index: confectionary, gum, bars, marshmallows, candy, cookies, snacks and popcorn.

In many ways the research is not surprising, but does it give you a new way of thinking about those treats? Naming them as treats or naught but nice is likely to mean you eat more of them. Naming them vice foods doesn't mean you can never eat them, but it may be that you will eat them less often.

157: The Obesity Depression Cycle

O besity is often accompanied by depression, and the two can interact, making each other worse.

A study by Floriana S. Luppino[323] and colleagues in *JAMA Psychiatry* concluded:

"We found bidirectional associations between depression and obesity: obese persons had a 55% increased risk of developing depression over time, whereas depressed persons had a 58% increased risk of becoming obese."

Weight gain doesn't usually happen immediately for people who are depressed. So, tackling depression early can ward off the further complications that being obese brings.

The American Psychological Association[324] offers this recommendation:

"... while treating obesity often helps decrease feelings of depression, weight loss is never successful if you remain burdened by stress and other negative feelings. You may have to work to resolve these issues first before beginning a weight-loss program."

158: Hot Food v Cold Food?

Science and technology educator Luis Villazon[325] says:

"Hot food does tend to make you feel full for longer, and this is because it increases the time it takes for your appetite to return. Freshly cooked food has more flavour because of the volatile organic compounds that are released, and this extra stimulation makes the food feel more satisfying than the same nutrients eaten cold.

"It's also much harder to bolt down hot food, and eating slowly signals to your brain that you are consuming a substantial meal – and so your brain suppresses your appetite for longer once you've finished your meal."

Culturally we also tend to see warm food as more satisfying. Researcher Amanda Pruski Yamim[326] advises adding a warm food item to a cold dish to increase the perceived feeling of fulness. Of course, you could also add a hot drink rather than a hot food item.

Maybe choosing a soup full of veggies would leave you feeling fuller than eating the same ingredients in a cold salad. Even so for your overall health it's important to eat some raw food.

159: Close The Menu

Y angjie Gu, Simona Botti, and David Faro from the London Business School (UK) published a study in the *Journal of Consumer Research*[327].

They looked at what happens when you provide consumers with a sense of closure. In this case it was the feeling that the decision was complete. They say:

"Subtle physical acts that symbolize closure can trigger choice closure and increase satisfaction."

In one of their studies, consumers were asked to choose one of twenty-four chocolates displayed on a tray covered by a lid. One group put the lid back on before eating the chocolate and the other group didn't.

In other studies, consumers chose an item from an extensive menu and either closed the menu or not before tasting the chosen item.

Consumers who closed the lid or the menu liked what they ate more than those who didn't perform an act of closure.

The study was about the level of satisfaction they experienced, but it seems likely that if you experience more satisfaction, you may eat less. Alternatively, you could enjoy it so much, you go back for more!

Next time you are faced with a box of chocolates put the lid on after you you've made your choice. Next time you're in a restaurant close the menu. See what happens to the amount you eat. Does this work as a strategy for eating less, but enjoying what you eat?

Many restaurants these days use menus that don't close. Is that because they want us to order more? Don't let them manipulate you in this way. Give the menu to the waiter or put it under your chair.

160: Benefits Of Being Overweight

Sometimes in order to gain control of your weight you have to address the benefits to you of being overweight. You may feel this is an outrageous thing for me to write – there are no benefits of being overweight!

But ask yourself this question honestly:

What benefits do I experience of being overweight?

Only you know the answer to this, but here are some possibilities:

- If you're overweight/obese, you don't have to deal with sexual attentions from other people.

- If you're overweight/obese, you don't need to confront your own sexuality.

- If you're overweight/obese you feel protected.

- If you're overweight/obese, you feel big/strong/important/imposing/noticed.

- If you're overweight/obese, another person will see how unhappy they have made you, and they will feel bad/do something about it.

- If you're overweight/obese, not much will be expected of you.

- If you're overweight/obese, it shows you won't be fat shamed by society. You're your own person.

- If you're overweight/obese, you won't feel like an outsider in your family.

Answering this question and dealing with the consequences can be your first step on a healthier relationship with food.

161: Justifying What You're Eating

D o you find yourself justifying what you're eating? For example:
  •I've had a hard day at work

- I deserve a treat now and then

- I didn't eat any breakfast

- I must have burned loads of calories when I was at my exercise class.

It could be that you're giving yourself an excuse to eat unhealthy food. Is it an excuse or a reason?

In my experience it's very rarely a reason. When you're hungry it's simple, you eat because you're hungry. You don't need any other reason.

There's usually something much better you can do to reward yourself or pick yourself up when you're making excuses to eat. See Hack 170.

162: Preventing Holiday Weight Gain

M
any people who are trying to gain control of their weight feel apprehensive about holidays or about celebrations such as Christmas and Thanksgiving. The way to get control of what feels like an uncontrollable situation is to plan ahead and to commit to certain practical strategies.

Much of the research has been done on helping people cope with national festive holidays rather than going away to another place on holiday.

A study by R C Baker[328] and D S Kirschenbaum published in Health Psychology found that participants who continued to self-monitor during a holiday period were less likely to gain weight. Self-monitoring included weighing themselves regularly. See Hack 134.

Psychologist Michelle vanDellen[329], University of Georgia, USA was one of the researchers looking at holiday weight gain. The research lasted between mid-November and January (14 weeks). Participants who weighed themselves every day and received graphical feedback of their weight changes either maintained or lost weight during the holiday season while participants who did not perform daily self-weighing gained weight. Associate professor vanDellen said:

"People are really sensitive to discrepancies or differences between their current selves and their standard or goal ... When they see that discrepancy, it tends to lead to behavioral change. Daily self-weighing ends up doing that for people in a really clear way."

Another study[330] published in the *Journal Of the Academy of Nutrition and Dietetics* found that maintaining physical exercise helped to reduce weight gain during the winter holiday season in the USA.

An article published in the *BMJ*[331] about a study designed to help prevent holiday weight gain concluded:

"A brief behavioural intervention involving regular self weighing, weight management advice, and information about the amount of physical activity required to expend the calories in festive foods and drinks prevented weight gain over the Christmas holiday period."

So once again we get self-weighing and physical activity being the key to managing this potentially difficult time.

It may feel unrealistic to hope for weight loss during the holiday season, although it's clear some people do manage this through weighing themselves and being active. Continuing (or starting) to weigh yourself regularly and finding ways to keep active will help you keep the weight off.

163: The Fat Brake

H ave you ever said (or heard someone else say): "Weight you put on quickly, you lose quickly"? Well, this appears to be true, but only for a short time.

Amanda Salis[332], Senior Research Fellow in the Boden Institute of Obesity, Nutrition, Exercise & Eating Disorders, University of Sydney (Australia) has written an interesting article in *The Conversation* on what she calls the "fat brake". And how it works post-holidays. She says:

"... whenever you consume more kilojoules than your body burns – think big, festive feasts and then sitting around for hours with your friends or relatives – your body activates a series of physiological processes that actually help you to reverse excess..."

"The most obvious sign of your fat brake is a reduction in your drive to eat. So in the aftermath of holiday overeating, if you're attentive to your body's hunger and satiety signals, you may not feel as drawn to as abundant or as rich foods. To make the most of this effect, it's important to not eat when you're not hungry – even if that means eating less than a weight-loss diet's allowance."

The crucial point here is that you need to follow what your body is telling you and not just return to your normal eating levels.

She says that eventually the fat brake deactivates. How long before this happens varies depending on how much excess weight you're carrying, how long you've been carrying it for, how much weight you've lost, and your genes. Often it is around 2 weeks.

If you don't act on the fat brake, it will still switch off. Then losing that extra weight will become more difficult. You have a small window of time to do this. Don't miss it.

The information about the fat brake can work in several ways. One is that you just pig out without any restraint in the knowledge that the fat brake will come into play. This is probably not a helpful way to think about it. Remember the fat brake doesn't work on its own. You have to recognise the reduction in your appetite and act on it.

Alternatively, you could stay determined not to over-indulge during the holiday season, knowing that there is this window of time if you don't succeed totally. Hopefully this will allow you to be less stressed as the holiday season approaches. This in itself will help you to control your eating. See Hack 41 Stress.

Look at Hack 162 Preventing Holiday Weight Gain to remind yourself what you need to do.

164: Active Holidays

Plan an active vacation/holiday - learn a new sport or go walking in a beautiful area. That way you get fitter and may not put on weight.

If being energetic doesn't suit you, what about going on a pilgrimage? People who undertake a pilgrimage follow a particular path with religious, spiritual or historical significance. I don't know of any research on what happens to people's weight on these trails, but it seems likely that they will either maintain or lose weight, as they walk and engage with something outside of themselves.

The best-known pilgrimage is probably the Camino de Santiago[333] in France and Spain, but it is definitely not the only one.

The Matador Network[334] suggests 7 less well-known pilgrimages (and there are others):

- St. Olav Ways, Norway

- Shikoku Pilgrimage, Japan

- Mount Kailash Kora, Tibet

- Camino del Norte, Spain

- Via Francigena, England, France, and Italy

- Baekdu-daegan Trail, South Korea

- The Abraham Path, The Middle East

165: Have A Script Ready

I hope that you have people who support you in your weight loss journey. But you're likely to have at least one person in your life who makes unhelpful comments.

If you're in this situation, spend some time working out responses, when you are not around them.

For example, if a family member is often tempting you with unhealthy food, try these responses:

- "Thanks, but I just ate"

- "It looks delicious, but not for me right now".

- "I'm trying to do something good for myself. Please support me in this."

- "If I keep eating all this sugary stuff, I'm depriving myself of a chance to be healthy."

- "I'm fine if you eat it in front of me. No worries."

The National Eating Disorders Association[335] (USA) says:

"You know those moments: when you can feel the topic of a conversation shifting into diet culture land, or when your Aunt So-and-so starts raving about her new diet, or how much weight your cousin Whats-his-name has gained or lost. It can be difficult to know what to say in the heat of the moment, so taking the time to come up with a few easy, quick comebacks can help you feel more confident:

- "You know I used to think about food that way too, but then I learned about

Intuitive Eating / how all foods are good foods/the dangers of diet culture/etc."

- "I'm actually learning to have a better relationship with food/my body, and that kind of talk is counterproductive"

- "The only kind of food you should feel guilty about eating is if you stole it from someone else!"

- "I think we should be focusing on all the things we're thankful for, rather than what our bodies look like"

- "I've actually stopped weighing myself and it's amazing how freeing it is"

"If you know that certain people always say the same things, or comment on certain things every year, use that knowledge and create your own comebacks!"

Even if you start eating more healthily, your family and friends may say that your food choices are weird or make some other negative comments. You may just have to ride these out, until the benefits of what you are eating begin to show them that you are making the right choices for you.

166: Friction Costs

Linda Bacon[336] (University of California, USA) and Lucy Aphramor (Coventry University, UK) have written an article in the *Nutrition Journal* arguing that the current emphasis on getting overweight and obese people to lose weight may be misguided. They write:

"Concern has arisen that this weight focus is not only ineffective at producing thinner, healthier bodies, but may also have unintended consequences, contributing to food and body preoccupation, repeated cycles of weight loss and regain, distraction from other personal health goals and wider health determinants, reduced self-esteem, eating disorders, other health decrement, and weight stigmatization and discrimination. This concern has drawn increased attention to the ethical implications of recommending treatment that may be ineffective or damaging."

Health at Every Size (HAES) focuses on health outcomes rather than weight outcomes. The HAES approach encourages body acceptance, intuitive eating (see hack 55) and finding enjoyable ways to stay active. The focus is not to lose weight but to become healthier. The authors say:

"Randomized controlled clinical trials indicate that a HAES approach is associated with statistically and clinically relevant improvements in physiological measures (e.g., blood pressure, blood lipids), health behaviors (e.g., eating and activity habits, dietary quality), and psychosocial outcomes (such as self-esteem and body image), and that HAES achieves these health outcomes more successfully than weight loss treatment and without the contraindications associated with a weight focus."

If you have tried many times to lose weight or keep weight off without long lasting success, the HAES approach is likely to be a healthier approach for you. Don't feel like you're giving up or that you're a failure or choosing something that's less powerful, the

HAES approach has been shown to be effective at helping people be healthier, without the obsession that a weight loss approach can bring.

The HAES approach can bring back some sanity if used wisely. But it's also important that you don't use it as an excuse to eat whatever you like.

Don't think you are concentrating on being healthy regardless of what you weigh while you eat high fat and high sugar foods. Being healthy whatever your size also means eating well and moving more.

167: It's My Genes!

If your parents are overweight or obese, how likely is it that you will be overweight or obese? There is a not a simple answer to this. A lot of the research in this area has been done on animals. It's very clear that we can't always extrapolate from animals to people.

It is possible you could weigh a lot because you have copied the eating habits of your family rather than having a genetic susceptibility. If your family way to reward success or console someone is to give high-calorie food, you are likely to struggle with your weight if you copy this.

The increase in obesity has been dramatic. It is highly unlikely that this is being driven by genetic mutations.

Harvard T H Chan School of Public Health[337] (USA) says:

"Genes influence every aspect of human physiology, development, and adaptation. Obesity is no exception. Yet relatively little is known regarding the specific genes that contribute to obesity and the scale of so-called "genetic environment interactions" the complex interplay between our genetic makeup and our life experiences."

They go on to say:

"What's increasingly clear from these early findings is that genetic factors identified so far make only a small contribution to obesity risk-and that our genes are not our destiny: Many people who carry these so-called "obesity genes" do not become overweight, and healthy lifestyles can counteract these genetic effects."

A study published in the *American Journal of Clinical Nutrition*[338] by Tiange Wang and colleagues looked at fruit and vegetable consumption. They found that improving fruit and vegetable intake reduces the genetic association with long-term weight gain.

The authors say:

"the beneficial effect was strongest for berries, citrus fruits, and green leafy vegetables, and for specific fruits and vegetables on the basis of fiber content and glycemic load."

See Hack 37 for more on the glycaemic load.

Dr Qibin Qi[339], Department of Nutrition at Harvard School of Public Health, confirmed that genes aren't all:

"In our study, a brisk one-hour daily walk reduced the genetic influence towards obesity, measured by differences in BMI by half. On the other hand, a sedentary lifestyle marked by watching television four hours a day increased the genetic influence by 50 percent."

John Mathers[340], Professor of Human Nutrition at Newcastle University (UK), has said of his study:

"You can no longer blame your genes. Our study shows that improving your diet and being more physically active will help you lose weight, regardless of your genetic makeup."

Harvard T H Chan School of Public Health[341] (USA) summarises the situation:

"Most people probably have some genetic predisposition to obesity, depending on their family history and ethnicity. Moving from genetic predisposition to obesity itself generally requires some change in diet, lifestyle, or other environmental factors."

In other words, genes are not, except in very rare people, a complete explanation of why you weigh more than you want to. Your diet and lifestyle play a big role too.

168: Coffee And Weight Loss

R egistered dietitian Katherine Zeratsky[342] writes on the Mayo Clinic (USA) website:

"Caffeine alone won't help you slim down. It may slightly boost weight-loss efforts or help prevent weight gain, but there's no solid evidence that caffeine consumption leads to noticeable weight loss."

Dr Derrick Johnston Alperet[343], Harvard T.H. Chan School of Public Health (USA) carried out a study in Singapore with Chinese, Malay or Asian-Indian participants. Subjects drank 4 cups of instant coffee a day for six months and saw a nearly 4% drop in overall body fat. He believes this is caused by an increase in metabolic rate.

He doesn't make it clear, but it seems that these participants did not normally drink coffee. If you're already drinking coffee, this intervention is unlikely to help.

Research[344] from the Centre for Nutrition, Exercise & Metabolism at the University of Bath (UK) found that drinking coffee to wake you up can have a negative effect on blood glucose (sugar) control.

Professor James Betts oversaw the research and said:

"Put simply, our blood sugar control is impaired when the first thing our bodies come into contact with is coffee especially after a night of disrupted sleep. We might improve this by eating first and then drinking coffee later if we feel we still feel the need it. Knowing this can have important health benefits for us all."

The whole area of coffee consumption is fraught with conflicting information. Studies have shown moderate coffee intake is beneficial for our health, and other studies have shown the opposite.

So, what to do? It's clear that heavy coffee drinking is detrimental to health. It seems unlikely that drinking coffee in moderation will have a noticeable effect on what you weigh. Following the University of Bath study, it's probably not good to reach for coffee before breakfast.

169: Health At Every Size

Linda Bacon[345] (University of California, USA) and Lucy Aphramor (Coventry University, UK) have written an article in the *Nutrition Journal* arguing that the current emphasis on getting overweight and obese people to lose weight may be misguided. They write:

"Concern has arisen that this weight focus is not only ineffective at producing thinner, healthier bodies, but may also have unintended consequences, contributing to food and body preoccupation, repeated cycles of weight loss and regain, distraction from other personal health goals and wider health determinants, reduced self-esteem, eating disorders, other health decrement, and weight stigmatization and discrimination. This concern has drawn increased attention to the ethical implications of recommending treatment that may be ineffective or damaging."

Health at Every Size (HAES) focuses on health outcomes rather than weight outcomes. The HAES approach encourages body acceptance, intuitive eating (see hack 55) and finding enjoyable ways to stay active. The focus is not to lose weight but to become healthier. The authors say:

"Randomized controlled clinical trials indicate that a HAES approach is associated with statistically and clinically relevant improvements in physiological measures (e.g., blood pressure, blood lipids), health behaviors (e.g., eating and activity habits, dietary quality), and psychosocial outcomes (such as self-esteem and body image), and that HAES achieves these health outcomes more successfully than weight loss treatment and without the contraindications associated with a weight focus."

If you have tried many times to lose weight or keep weight off without long lasting success, the HAES approach is likely to be a healthier approach for you. Don't feel like you're giving up or that you're a failure or choosing something that's less powerful, the HAES approach has been shown to be effective at helping people be healthier, without the obsession that a weight loss approach can bring.

The HAES approach can bring back some sanity if used wisely. But it's also important that you don't use it as an excuse to eat whatever you like.

Don't think you are concentrating on being healthy regardless of what you weigh while you eat high fat and high sugar foods. Being healthy whatever your size also means eating well and moving more.

170: Rewarding Yourself

One common way of rewarding ourselves is with food:

- •I've spent ages cleaning the kitchen/ doing my tax return/being patient with my mum, so I deserve a little reward. I think I'll have a bar of chocolate.

- Now that I've joined the gym, I can have a cake.

This is fine occasionally. If you do it regularly, your weight is likely to increase and your health suffer from these high calorie, unhealthy foods.

Some people reward themselves with alcohol:

- I've had a hard day at work, so I'll open a bottle of wine (or two).

- My health problems are really getting me down, a large gin will cheer me up.

- I've finally tidied up the house, so now I can chill out with some beer.

Occasionally this is fine, but it can turn from an occasional thing to a dependence on alcohol.

Rewarding ourselves can be an important part of doing things successfully. It's good to celebrate achieving goals, and important markers along the way to our biggest goals.

On your weight loss journey or your maintenance journey, you will want to reward yourself:

Robert Taibbi[346] writes in *Psychology Today*:

"At some point in your efforts to break a habit, you reach a point where you go: Why am I bothering to struggle with this? You feel discouraged, you feel you are emotionally making your life seemingly harder and that there is little payoff.

"This is normal, the low point in the process, and you need to keep your eyes on the prize. But you also need to make sure you build in a payoff."

So here are 25 suggestions for rewarding yourself without turning to food or alcohol:

1. Listen to the whole of a favourite music album without doing anything else at the same time.

2. Buy some fruit or vegetables that you wouldn't normally buy because they are too expensive.

3. Buy something small that you've always wanted.

4. Relax in the park or at the beach.

5. Visit a local museum or art gallery.

6. See a movie.

7. Meet up with a friend you really like but haven't seen for a while.

8. Watch a box set.

9. Extra cuddle time with someone you love.

10. Go someplace you've never been before.

11. Search for new music.

12. Indulge in a guilty pleasure, such as watching some trashy tv or reading a gossip magazine.

13. Schedule a beauty session.

14. Take time for a hobby.

15. Take a nap.

16. Stay in your pyjamas all day.

17. Have a sauna.

18. Get your groceries delivered rather than going to the shop.

19. Have time without the internet.

20. Go look at the stars.

21. Use a taxi rather than public transport for one of your normal journeys.

22. Have a massage.

23. Play with your neighbour's dog.

24. Buy yourself some flowers.

25. Add some essential oils to a bath and have a long, leisurely soak.

It's unlikely that you'll like all of these. Start with this list but remove some and add other things that will give you a sense of reward.

171: Weight Loss Apps

In 2016 experts[347] from the University of Sydney ranked weight loss apps.

After examining 800 apps for the study, researchers selected 28 apps that were weight management-specific and allowed for logging food intake. Each app was used for five days and assessed against a range of quality measures:

- the credibility of their information source

- the accuracy and coverage of scientific information

- the inclusion of enhanced features (like barcode scanners) usability

- their likelihood of changing health behaviours.

Juliana Chen, a dietitian involved in the research said:

"Make sure the app comes from a credible source, and that health professionals have been involved in developing it. We found that a large number of weight loss apps are developed by people with little scientific understanding of what would support weight loss.

"Choose an app which includes techniques for changing behaviour – these were generally the apps which rated the best in our evaluation. Apps that include more motivational components, such as points, levels, feedback, rewards and challenges, are more likely to lead to changes in behaviour.

"Check to see if the information provided in the app matches up with reliable sources on healthy eating, such as the Australian Dietary Guidelines."

She goes on to say:

"Using an app to support weight loss can be helpful for people who want to get a better idea of the amount of food and kilojoules they are eating each day.

"However, you need to be a highly motivated person to maintain the food logging over a prolonged period of time. Many people find the process becomes tedious, and their engagement with the app drops off.

"What leads to more effective weight loss is using an app in conjunction with weight loss counselling from a health professional who can help you with goal setting and identifying barriers and enablers to follow your plan. This kind of personally tailored advice and feedback unfortunately just isn't available in an app."

Of the devices studied they found Noom Weight Loss Coach[348] (Noom Inc) the most likely to change behaviour and assist weight loss.

But remember this study was done in 2016 and the apps were only studied for 5 days by experts who don't necessarily need to lose weight themselves.

A 2020 study[349] in the journal *Frontiers in Endocrinology* concluded:

Overall, evidence suggests that mobile applications may be useful as low-intensity approaches or adjuncts to conventional weight management strategies. However, there is insufficient evidence to support their use as stand-alone intensive approaches to weight management.

A study in 2021[350] published in the *Journal of Internet Medical Research* concluded:

"Motivating users to use an app over time could help them better achieve their nutrition goals. Although user reviews generally showed positive opinions and ratings of the apps, developers should pay more attention to users' technical problems and inform users about expected payments, along with their refund and cancellation policies, to increase user loyalty."

All in all, the researchers are saying that using an app is probably not enough on its own to help you lose weight, but it may be beneficial as part of an overall strategy. The main problem is some people get fed up of inputting data on what they are eating.

172: Food Density

F ood density, also called calorie density, is a measure of the number of calories in a given weight of food. Chocolate has a higher density than lettuce, because it has more calories in the same weight than lettuce does.

Barbara J Rolls and colleagues from the US Pennsylvania State University looked at the effect of eating low energy-dense soup. They published their findings in Obesity Research[351]:

"On an energy-restricted diet, consuming two servings of low energy-dense soup daily led to 50% greater weight loss than consuming the same amount of energy as high energy-dense snack food. Regularly consuming foods that are low in energy density can be an effective strategy for weight management."

One way of decreasing the energy density of a meal is to add pureed vegetables. In one study published in the American Journal of Clinical Nutrition[352] participants reduced their consumption by around 350 kcal a day without feeling hungrier.

Participants were fed a standard version (rated as 100%) or one rated at 85% and one rated at 75% energy density. Those eating the 85% density reduced their calorie consumption by around 200 kcal a day and those on the 75% regime had a reduced consumption of around 350 kcal. Over time this would mount up to a significant weight loss and without feeling hungry all the time.

The idea of adding pureed vegetables to your meals may not be appealing, but there are other options that reduce the overall density of your meal.

Julie E Flood and Barbara J Rolls[353] of Pennsylvania State University (USA) found that consuming soup at the beginning of a meal can significantly reduce subsequent entrée/main course intake, as well as total energy intake at the meal.

Another study[354] showed that eating low energy-dense salads at the beginning of a meal led to fewer calories being consumed overall. Low energy dense salads are ones containing lots of vegetables such as salad leaves, cucumber, tomatoes. High density salads, which won't work to decrease your overall calorie intake, might contain pasta or m eat.

So, the takeaway from this is to eat more foods that are less dense. Less dense foods generally contain more water and/or fibre.

Fast foods and snacks tend to be high density. Vegetables and fruit are usually low density. Increasing your intake of fruit and vegetables has lots of other health benefits too.

The US Centers For Disease Control[355] (CDC) in a booklet called "More Volume, Fewer Calories" offers this advice:

- Add water to your meals via soups and stews

- Drink smaller portions of fruit juice by adding water

- Add fruit to your meal to increase water and fibre

- Begin your meal with a salad.

- Add legumes (beans/pulses) to your meals

- Use whole grains

- Use nuts in small quantities

173: Salads

Salads are often seen as a mainstay of any weight loss diet, but more important than that they are part of a healthy diet. Sadly, lots of people say they don't like salads. They often find them boring. If this is you, let me see if I can change your mind.

I regularly post vegan salad pics on Instagram (@thrivingjane[356]), and people often comment how tasty and interesting they look. Even non-vegans will say this!

This is a vegan salad recipe for people like me who want to eat well, but they aren't good at the planning.

There isn't, of course, one vegan salad that is the best. It depends on your preferences, what you have available, now hungry you are. The perfect vegan salad will be different depending on how you answer these questions.

Before I start to make a salad, I ask myself a few questions:

- What have I got available?

- How hungry am I?

- Do I want a chopped salad, a regular tossed salad or a salad of separated ingredients?

So, let's look at each of these in turn.

What have I got available?

I'm not that organised when it comes to eating. For my salad I generally open the fridge door and see what's there. I do occasionally cook extra rice or potatoes or quinoa for an evening meal so that I have something left over for the next day's salad, but that's as organised as I get!

Everything comes out from the fridge on to the workbench. As I cast my eyes round what is available, a combination will sometimes immediately jump out at me, but sometimes it gets built bit by bit. I don't necessarily use everything I have available.

Cold veggies can be unappetising, but fried with some spices (cumin, coriander, chilli, curry powder) so they have crispy bits, they make a great addition to a salad. Either prepare these first and allow to cool or do them last and pile on top still sizzling for contrast and interest. You can top this topping with some black onion seeds or black sesame seeds to add extra interest and nutrition.

Left over risotto crumbled up or cold pasta chopped can make interesting additions too.

I also try to keep some jars of salad ingredients available. For example, olives, artichokes, sun dried tomatoes make great additions to a salad and will keep for some time in a fridge.

How hungry am I?

What can I put in salad to fill me up? If I'm really hungry, I want to make a grain the starting point of my salad. That's where the rice or quinoa come in. If I don't have them, it may be a salad with a hunk of bread or some corn chips or some crisps (potato chips).

What sort of salad do I want?

I often make a salad where each ingredient has its own place on the plate. These are brought together by a splash of olive oil and vinegar, some chilli jam or one of the many vegan salad dressings you can buy now. This is definitely the quickest way to make the salad. I go for lots of colour and try to put contrasting colours next to each other. This makes it really pleasing to the eye. Black olives next to the vibrant red of tomatoes, salad leaves next to some grated carrot. If my salad ingredients don't give me these vibrant contrasting colours, I know I'm missing a vital component of healthy food, eating the ra inbow.

A chopped salad takes more work but is great as a change. You need a sharp knife. and chop most things.

Don't just chop! Yes, that's right. If you chop everything, the ingredients tend to clump together. So better chop some (salad leaves, peppers, tomatoes, etc.), slice some (cucumber, celery, baby tomatoes, etc.) and grate some (carrot, celeriac, courgette/zucchini, etc.) and leave some whole (capers, beans, pumpkin seeds etc.). This increases the textures, so is more interesting and more pleasing to look at.

Use lots of different ingredients and lots of different colours - not only are you getting a wide range of vitamins, minerals and phytochemicals, but it's also hugely appealing to the eye.

Then I just toss everything together and add some dressing. Chopped salads are great for when I want to take it with me to eat later. They also help you eat more salad, if you put it on your plate ready tossed.

The third option is to toss the salad without chopping, I generally don't like this unless I'm just making a simple green salad. A salad with heavier ingredients doesn't toss well.

What can I put in my salad instead of meat? So, as I'm vegan, I'm not going to put meat or fish or eggs or cheese in my salad, but there are lots of other things.

Sometimes it will be a burger, either homemade or bought, with the salad piled up by its side.

I might have lentils or beans – chickpeas or puy lentils are my favourites. I sometimes dress these with oil and vinegar, a bought salad dressing or a dollop of mayonnaise. Gram flour pancakes or fried tofu will take the place of that burger sometimes.

I often have nuts in my salad, because I love them. Happily, there is mounting evidence we should eat at least one portion of nuts a day. (See Hack 102) I don't usually chop them, even when I'm having a chopped salad! Almonds and cashew nuts work well. Salted peanuts make a great addition too. And I adore walnuts with avocado or whole lentils.

I love seeds – they're tasty and packed with nutrition. My favourites are sunflower seeds and pumpkin seeds. Sometimes I toast them, by adding them to a hot dry pan and cooking them quickly till they start popping. Then I might add some tamari or just leave them as they are.

I also have some hero salad ingredients. These are ingredients that just lift a salad to a whole new level. For me there are three that I often turn to:

Mint – has to be fresh and chopped – sometimes mixed in with the salad and sometimes added on top. See Hack 92 for information about mint's role as an appetite suppressant.

Capers – particularly good with a chopped salad. You can buy these in jars, and they keep well in the fridge.

Preserved lemons – a personal favourite that I add to all sorts of things - they're great with chilli! My partner John hates them, you may too, but do give them a try. Again, they come in jars. Take out a piece of lemon, wash to remove most of the salt and chop finely.

I hope this has given you some ideas about how to make the best salad – one you will enjoy and will feed you with the nutrients you need to live a vibrant life.

174: Eat More Veggies

R egistered Dietitian Anne Myers-Wright[357] says:

"Research has shown that serving a variety of vegetables at each meal (rather than just including one on your plate) can increase vegetable intake. This could be as simple as adding one or two extra types of vegetables each time you eat – for example, instead of serving broccoli alone, why not try broccoli, baby corn and roasted cherry tomatoes? Eating the same vegetables for most meals can become boring and bland for our taste buds. If you can, mix things up and try something your palette hasn't had in a w hile."

This approach is supported by Hack 08.

She also says:

"If you find that you're not eating much veg with your meals because you don't know where to begin with how to cook and add them into your meal or you don't have much time – then don't be afraid to use frozen vegetables."

The Heart Research Institute UK[358] says:

"Vegetables are the cornerstone of a healthy diet. If you make them the primary component of your meals, you maximise your nutrient intake and decrease your energy intake. For managing your weight long term, this is one of the most important things you can do."

An article[359] in the academic journal *Nutrients* reviewing various studies concluded that:

"... increased intake of FV [fruit and vegetables] to recommended levels of intake is a chief contributor to successful weight loss in women"

175: Green Tea

It's a lovely idea that drinking green tea can help you effortlessly lose weight. But what is the evidence?

A review of the research published in the *Canadian Pharmacists Journal*[360] concluded:

"The ability of green tea preparations to help with weight loss has been evaluated in a Cochrane Systematic Review that included 14 RCTs [randomised controlled trials]. Those in the green tea group lost on average 0.2 to 3.5 kg more than those in the control group over 12 weeks. In most studies, the weight loss was not statistically significant."

The studies were using a green tree extract rather than giving people green tea to drink.

Much of the work showing the beneficial effects of green tea was undertaken on people who probably aren't like you: people who were not overweight or who were highly active[361].

Sometimes the supplement being tested included other substances such as caffeine. Some of the studies are based on animals, so cannot be reliably carried over to people.

If you enjoy green tea or want to drink it for other health reasons, please do. But don't rely on it to solve your weight problems.

176: Second Helpings

If you always want a second helping, make your first helping smaller, so that you can have that second helping without putting on weight.

177: Weight Loss Surgery

The UK NHS website[362] says:

"Weight loss surgery, also called bariatric or metabolic surgery, is sometimes used as a treatment for people who are very obese.

"It can lead to significant weight loss and help improve many obesity-related conditions, such as type 2 diabetes or high blood pressure.

"But it's a major operation and in most cases should only be considered after trying to lose weight through a healthy diet and exercise."

The website goes on to say:

"Weight loss surgery can achieve dramatic weight loss, but it's not a cure for obesity on its own.

"You'll need to commit to making permanent lifestyle changes after surgery to avoid putting weight back on."

Weight loss surgery should always be viewed as a last resort. You need to be eating a healthy diet whether or not you have a weight problem or have had weight loss surgery.

178: Alpha-Lipoic Acid

Alpha-lipoic acid (ALA) is found in foods such as red meat, carrots, beets, spinach, broccoli, and potatoes. But the research has predominantly been done using supplements.

Suat Kucukgoncu[363] and colleagues from Yale University (USA) looked at research in this area in 2017. They identified 10 articles on randomised, double-blind, placebo-controlled studies involving ALA.

They concluded:

"ALA treatment showed small, yet significant short-term weight loss compared to placebo. Further research is needed to examine the effect of different doses and the long-term benefits of ALA on weight management."

Researchers[364] from Oregon State University (USA) and Oregon Health & Science University (USA) analysed the effects of 24 weeks of daily, 600-milligram doses of lipoic acid supplements on 31 people, with a similarly sized control group receiving a placebo.

Balz Frei, one of the researchers, said:

"The data clearly showed a loss in body weight and body fat in people taking lipoic acid supplements ... Particularly in women and in the heaviest participants."

Another review of the literature by Mahdi Vajdi[365] and Mahdieh Abbasalizad Farhangi of Tabriz University of Medical Sciences (Iran) in 2021 concluded:

"ALA treatment significantly reduced BMI ... While the association of ALA treatment on WC [waist circumference] is dependent to the duration of the study.

Alpha-lipoic acid supplements certainly seem to be producing results. But do remember if you decide to take this supplement, buy from a reputable supplier and do not exceed the stated dose.

Also remember that taking alpha-lipoic acid is almost certainly not enough on its own. It's not a substitute for eating well and taking exercise.

179: Visualisation

There seems to be lots of anecdotal evidence about losing weight though visualisation, but the scientific evidence is much harder to come by. Visualisation can be about how you would look and/or about how you would feel.

Researchers[366] from the University of Plymouth (UK) and Queensland University of Technology (Australia) found that people who used Functional Imagery Training (FIT) lost an average of five times more weight than those using talking therapy alone. This is a massive result.

FIT visualisation is multi-sensory, so not just relying on vision. The lead researcher, Dr Linda Solbrig, explained:

"We started with taking people through an exercise about a lemon. We asked them to imagine seeing it, touching it, juicing it, drinking the juice and juice accidently squirting in their eye, to emphasise how emotional and tight to our physical sensations imagery is. From there we are able to encourage them to fully imagine and embrace their own goals. Not just 'imagine how good it would be to lose weight' but, for example, 'what would losing weight enable you to do that you can't do now? What would that look/sound/smell like?', and encourage them to use all of their senses."

Check out Hack 119 Feel Rather Than Achieve for some related information.

Gemma Ossolinski[367] and colleagues from Australian universities studied the effect of computer-generated images on weight loss.

Participants received general healthy lifestyle information at recruitment and were weighed at 4-weekly intervals for 24 weeks. All participants were given a hard copy future self-image either at recruitment (early image) or after 8 weeks (delayed image). The image was generated using the app Future Me. The delayed-image group did consistently better in terms of weight loss. One in five participants in the delayed-image group completing the 24-week intervention achieved a clinically significant weight loss, having received only future self-images and general lifestyle advice.

This is worth trying if you have access to this app or a similar one. It clearly doesn't make a significant difference for everyone, but it works for some people. Remember it's most effective to generate the image after a delay. In the case of this research it was 8 weeks, although the study only tested this time delay, so we don't know if even better results would be obtained with a different delay.

Bärbel Knäuper[368], a psychologist at McGill University (Canada) asked 177 students to set themselves the goal of consuming more fruit for a period of seven days. All the students in the study ended up consuming more fruit over the course of the week than they had beforehand. But those who made a concrete plan, wrote it down and also visualised how they were going to carry out the action increased their fruit consumption twice as much as those who simply set out to eat more fruit without visualizing and planning how they were going to do it.

Bärbel Knäuper said:

"These kinds of visualization techniques are borrowed from sports psychology. "Athletes do lots of work mentally rehearsing their performances before competing and it's often very successful. So we thought having people mentally rehearse how they were going to buy and eat their fruit should make it more likely that they would actually do it. And this is exactly what happened."

There's a lot more research needed in this area, but it's clear that visualisation in all its different forms can work well for some people.

180: Meal Frequency

E ating lots of small meals has become popular. Proponents argue that it helps maintain blood sugar levels and so stops you wanting to binge. Others argue that you should stick to the traditional three meals a day or do some form of intermittent fasting (see Hack 97).

So, which is best?

Mia Syn[369], a registered dietitian nutritionist, sums this up nicely when she writes:

"There are many different perspectives on the optimal frequency of eating, in general, and specifically for weight loss. While there is a lot of helpful research on this topic, one "right" or "best" way of timing your meals that will result in weight loss and/or maintenance has not emerged. This is likely because there are so many variables, from the types of foods eaten and each body's metabolism and nutritional needs to a person's ability to adhere to a diet plan.

"In fact, while there are many studies that show eating more frequent meals leads to a lower risk of obesity and health complications (such as diabetes and cardiovascular disease), there are also many showing the opposite. Additionally, what happens during a controlled study may not always reflect eating in the real world.

"There are many eating plan options ... You might simply need to experiment to find the right meal timing for you - one that you feel good about and that you can maintain without burdensome effort."

So once again it's over to you – you need to be the scientist in your life and find what works for you. Are you better off with multiple small meals?

181: What Can You Control?

It's easy to focus on the problems – the partner who always buys lots of irresistible treats or the lack of time to plan meals. If you do this, it's difficult to do anything. You are likely to put on weight and feel bad about yourself.

So, focus on what <u>you</u> can control. This is, of course, different for different people. Ignore for the time being the things that you feel you can't control and optimize the things you can control.

Caroline M. Apovian, MD and Judith Korner, MD, PhD write in the *Journal of Clinical Endocrinology & Metabolism*[370]:

"Most importantly, focus on what you can control. You can control what you eat and whether you go for a walk. But you can't control how fast you lose weight. If you find that your plan isn't working, it doesn't mean you've failed. Instead, it means you should change your plan. Find a plan that works for you."

182: Not Enough Time

O ne of the things that can get in the way of a healthy lifestyle is the feeling that you don't have enough time. You don't have time to prepare food in advance, to cook healthily or to take exercise.

"If you don't make time for your wellness, you'll be forced to make time for your illness." I've seen this quote attributed to various people. It's unclear who first said it, but it's also clear that it's likely to be true.

Even if you know this to be true, it can be difficult to do the things you know you should do when you have so many things on your to-do list.

I find using the method attributed to US President Dwight D. Eisenhower. works well. It has since been popularised by Stephen Covey in his book *First Things First*.

Tasks can be divided into 4 categories:

Quadrant 1: Important And Urgent

Activities that we have to do and so we make time for them. If you're a parent, you may have to pick your child up at a certain time. You may have a work project with an urgent deadline. It can feel like we are being very productive. Some of these tasks can be very exciting and make us feel important.

Quadrant 2: Important But Not Urgent

Activities that are important to your core values and your vision but do not have any urgency attached to them. Activities such as spending time with your family, taking exercise, relaxing, long-term planning, anticipating and preventing problems, self-development activities, etc. fall into this category. We intend to do these things, but often get involved in activities in the other quadrants instead.

Quadrant 3: Unimportant But Urgent

Activities that other people might feel are important, but they are not important to us because they do not involve our core values and vision. Some people spend a lot of time in this area because they want to please, or not upset other people. It can involve answering emails, although some emails are, of course, important. It can mean helping solve the problem of your children or other people when they could easily solve them themselves. Being in this area a lot eventually makes you feel powerless and dissatisfied.

Quadrant 4: Unimportant And Not Urgent

These are activities that use up a lot of time, but do not achieve anything. Note that genuine leisure activities are not included in this category, because they are important, so they are in Quadrant 2. Activities in this category include mindlessly surfing the web and watching a lot of television.

So where does healthy eating and weight management fit in all this? It's clearly Important But Not Urgent. If you don't make yourself a salad lunch to take to work today, nothing very much will happen. It has no urgency. If you have a fast-food takeaway tonight rather than cooking a healthy meal from scratch, the consequences are small.

This is the reason why so many Important But Not Urgent activities don't happen. An individual event has very little effect. It's the cumulative effect that causes the problem.

How to use this information? You can list your activities in each quadrant. Is it possible to do less in quadrant 4, so you have more time for quadrant 2?

Another way is to be aware of this matrix on a daily basis. Whenever you feel overwhelmed or that your healthy lifestyle is slipping, ask yourself: what quadrant 2 activity can I do to make things better for myself? You probably have a lot of quadrant 2 activities that won't take a lot of time.

Alternatively, commit yourself to doing 3 (say) quadrant 2 activities each day.

Another useful approach is to look at the things you always have time for, no matter what. Why do you commit to those things and not healthy eating? Does it help to reflect on why those things are important?

Living a healthy lifestyle is about prioritising it because it's important to you, regardless of how busy you are.

183: Create A Ritual

Yep, create a ritual, any ritual! Let me explain.

Francesca Gino[371], a behavioural scientist and Tandon Family Professor of Business Administration at Harvard Business School conducted research using meaningless, but precise, rituals. She explains:

In one study she recruited undergraduate women who already had a goal of losing weight.

"We told half of them to be mindful about their food consumption for the next five days. We taught the other half a three-step pre-eating ritual and told them to complete it every time they ate something.

"... participants who enacted the pre-eating ritual consumed fewer calories (about 1,424 calories for each day, on average) as compared to those who simply were mindful about their eating (who consumed about 1,648). Those who performed the ritual also ate less fat and less sugar."

You are probably now wondering what this miracle ritual was.

Professor Gino explains the ritual instructions that were given to the participants:

"First, cut your food into pieces before you eat it. Second, rearrange the pieces so that they are perfectly symmetric on your plate. That is, get the right half of your plate to look exactly the same as the left half of your plate. Finally, press your eating utensil against the top of your food three times. In order to be in the study, you must do the three steps of this ritual each time you eat."

The professor did other experiments with other participants using other mindless, but precise, rituals.

But why would it work?

Professor Gino says:

"Following a series of steps over and over again, which happens when we use rituals, requires some good self-discipline. So, we reasoned, when we see ourselves engaging in a ritual, we code that behavior as a sign that we are people with self-control. And thanks to that self-control, we choose the apple (or carrot) over the chocolate and thus reduce our caloric intake."

The exact nature of the ritual itself was not important. It was having the ritual and doing it before they ate anything.

There are several possible problems with this study.

Professor Gino says:

"Interestingly, at the end of the study, our participants said they thought the ritual was not very helpful and reported they were unlikely to continue it."

Reading this last sentence may mean you won't try it because the participants didn't think it was helpful. Of course, the answer is that it did help. On average the participants using the ritual consumed 200 calories a day less without being aware that they had made any change to what they ate. They also ate more healthily. Hacks that mean that you eat less without being aware of it are just the sort of hacks most people are looking for!

Professor Gino cautions:

"It is important to note that rituals like the ones we created and used in our research can be taken too far. When a repeated set of actions that restrict food consumption start to become mindlessly followed, as by habit, they can lead to problematic behaviors such as eating disorders, research finds. But undertaken conscientiously and carefully, such practices can also promote well-being."

Finally, this research was only over a short time. The study mentioned here, happened over five days. We do not know what would happen if you carried the ritual on for weeks or months.

But, taking all that into account, it's definitely worth trying this and seeing if you find it helpful. And remember you don't have to use the ritual suggested here. Also remember that it doesn't have to be meaningful in itself. It's doing it every time before you eat that makes the connection and makes it work. It makes you feel that you have self-control and self-discipline. Those are feelings that are important if you want to gain weight control.

184: Spot Reduction

Spot reduction refers to the idea that fat in a certain area of the body can be targeted for reduction through exercise of specific muscles in that area.

Health and Fitness Expert Jessica Matthews[372] writes about spot reduction on the website of The American Council On Exercise. She writes:

"It is important to understand that "spot reducing" is not possible. The concept of spot reducing is based on the flawed notion that it is possible to "burn off" fat from a specific part of the body by selectively exercising that area. However, numerous studies have refuted this claim."

She goes on to say:

"Arguably the most compelling evidence refuting the myth of spot reduction comes from a study conducted at the University of Massachusetts in the mid-1980s. In this investigation, 13 male subjects participated in a vigorous abdominal exercise training program for 27 days. Each participant in the study was required to perform a total of 5,000 sit-ups over the course of the research project. Fat biopsies were obtained from the subjects' abdomens, buttocks and upper backs before and after the exercise program ... the results of the study revealed that fat decreased similarly at all three sites — not just in the abdominal region. These findings may help explain one reason why spot reducing sometimes appears to work. If the caloric expenditure is sufficient enough, it will cause fat from the entire body to be reduced, including a particular target area."

If spot reduction was possible, these participants would have lost more weight on their abdomens, rather than all over their bodies.

Yet don't despair, you may be able to tone an area with specific exercises, so that it looks like you have less fat there. Also, by building toned muscle in your arms and shoulders, it can make your hips seem visually less large.

185: Radical Change

Many diet trends and diet books are founded on the idea of radical change. It is the idea that with the right mind set and goals you can change your life completely in a short amount of time.

The beach-body-in-12-weeks-approach offers the idea of a dramatic change. If you don't succeed, it's because you didn't commit enough, you ate too much, exercised too little. You failed.

James Clear[373] thinks the idea of radical change is a myth:

"The myth of radical change and overnight success is pervasive in our culture. Experts say things like, "The biggest mistake most people make in life is not setting goals high enough." Or they tell us, "If you want massive results, then you have to take massive action.""

He goes on to explain why this doesn't work for most people:

"On the surface, these phrases sound inspiring. What we fail to realize, however, is that any quest for rapid growth contradicts every stabilizing force in our lives. Remember, the natural tendency of life is to find stability. Anytime equilibrium is lost, the system is motivated to restore it.

"If you step too far outside the bounds of your normal performance, then nearly all of the forces in your life will be screaming to get you back to equilibrium. If you take massive action, then you quickly run into a massive roadblock."

This doesn't mean we can't change. It does mean that for most of the time change comes in a slower more measured way.

Janes Clear goes on to say:

"... the best way to achieve a new level of equilibrium is not with radical change, but through small wins each day.

"This is the great paradox of behavior change. If you try to change your life all at once, you will quickly find yourself pulled back into the same patterns as before. But if you merely focus on changing your normal day, you will find your life changes naturally as a side effect."

186: Weight Loss?

We all talk about weight loss, but losing things is usually considered a cause for dismay.

Maybe you need to change the phrase to something more positive. Try:

- Weight control

- Appetite management

- Slimness gain

- Shape regain

- Health regain

- Positive weight mentality

- Body harmony

- Self-esteem regain

Maybe none of these work for you, but I'm sure you can think of others that will.

187: Your Comfort Zone

What's your comfort zone? What are you like in your comfort zone? You may well have to move out of your comfort zone in order to lose weight and keep it off.

You may have to put yourself first more often. You may need to face up to what you've done to your body. You may need to confront shame and anger.

Your comfort zone may not feel that comfortable, but it probably feels a lot more comfortable than the risky idea of moving out of it.

John Colbert of www.corporate-edge.com.au[374] writes:

"The problem is that while we remain in our comfort zones, generally we're not learning or growing as people. Being too scared to step out of your comfort zone in the long term can prevent you from achieving your goals or improving your level [of] happiness.

"Growth is uncomfortable – so if we want to achieve growth in any area of life, we need to get comfortable with feeling uncomfortable."

He offers 4 key insights:

- Remember there's a first time for everything

- Acknowledge the challenge

- Think of the benefits

- Accept it's okay to fail

He writes:

"If things don't go the way you want, think about what you can learn from it and start the process again. Don't ever lose sight of the fact that this is exactly what personal growth is supposed to feel like... If you can do small things often enough and for long enough, your comfort zone will expand, and you'll find yourself quickly growing as a person."

So, expand your comfort zone bit by bit and develop better weight control.

188: The Story You Tell Yourself

Talking to a personal trainer at the gym set me thinking about the way we see ourselves. The way we see ourselves is often an important reason why we fail or succeed.

Mat, the PT, has had major knee surgery and for some time was using crutches. Now he's walking on his own, but he is still a long way from being the active athlete he has been. That all lies ahead in the future.

When someone who is used to training regularly stops, they often put on a lot of weight. They keep eating like they did when they needed all that food to fuel their activity, their muscle repair and muscle growth. They often feel bored and frustrated that they can't train. That often leads to eating comfort food.

I remarked to Mat that he'd done well not to put on weight. He replied:

"I'm a nutrition coach, so of course I know how to manage my weight."

He spoke as if it wasn't difficult. He knew the sort of person he was, so he knew he could do it. And he had.

When challenges occur in your lives, the result is in part determined by the sort of person you believe you are. It is affected by the story you tell yourself about yourself.

So, how do you see yourself? This is in part determined by how you were brought up and what your parents said to you. See Hack 141 for more on this.

It's interesting how as adults we let one event determine how we view ourselves. It's a bit like our attitude to restaurants. We can go to a restaurant many times and have wonderful food. Then we go once and have a bad experience. Many of us will stop going to that restaurant, because we don't want to be disappointed again. We forget all the great meals and focus on the one bad meal.

Similarly, we concentrate on the one time we forgot what we were saying when we were giving a public lecture. We remember the time we played appalling golf, not all the times we did really well, and everything just flowed. We keep replaying that stupid mistake, rather than all the times we succeeded.

We remember all the time we've given into temptation and pigged out on food. We remember regaining the weight we've worked so hard to lose.

We become defined by these failures. So instead of thinking that we've given some great talks, played some great games or had great success socially, we define ourselves by the failures. We forget that we ate healthily for several weeks at a time.

If you find yourself doing this, take some time and write a list of your successes. They can be small things. They don't have to be big enterprises or amazing breakthroughs. All the daily wins add up to the person you are. Write them down and read them or go through them in your mind when you see yourself defined by your failures.

They don't even need to be about weight management and healthy eating. Success in any area of your life can help you feel you can be successful in anything you want to achieve.

You may need to develop a whole new way of seeing yourself to gain control of your weight and how you see your body. That isn't going to happen overnight. It will take work to achieve it. Start now by asking yourself: what sort of person am I? Does that sort of person lose weight and keep it off?

189: Failure

Thomas Edison invented the electric light bulb. He once said, "I have not failed 10,000 times - I've successfully found 10,000 ways that will not work."

Don't despair if you've been struggling for years to lose weight - you now know lots of ways that don't work. Think about the ways that you've tried – do they give you any clues about what might work?

Franklin D Roosevelt said:

"It is common sense to take a method and try it. If it fails, admit it frankly and try another. But above all, try something."

Mary Pickford said:

There is always another chance ... This thing we call 'failure' is not the falling down, but the staying down."

Business coach Zig Ziglar remarked:

"Understand that failure is an event, not a person."

190: Hope

Harvard T H Chan School of Public Health[375] (USA) says:

"Losing as little as 5 to 10 percent of body weight offers meaningful health benefits to people who are obese, even if they never achieve their "ideal" weight, and even if they only begin to lose weight later in life."

Losing a few kilograms in weight almost halves people's risk of developing Type 2 diabetes, according to a large scale research study, Norfolk Diabetes Prevention Study[376], the largest diabetes prevention research study in the world in the last 30 years. The NDPS clinical trial ran over eight years and involved more than 1,000 people with prediabetes at high risk of developing Type 2 diabetes.

Final Thoughts

T his book is about hope – giving you ideas and insights to help you achieve something that you want so much.

Some of the research cited in the book talks about how many people put weight back on. That can be depressing to read. But remember the traditional ways to lose weight focus on calorie reduction. The vast majority of people who have lost weight did it that way – their weight regain was almost inevitable. Only now are we beginning to understand that this isn't the long-term solution for most people.

More and more research and experience are showing that you need to concentrate on eating a healthy diet, with lots of veggies and fruit. You need to think about eating low density foods with lots of water and fibre in them. You need to minimise sugar and fast foods.

You also need to look at how you eat and when you eat. You need to unpack the role emotions and stress play in your weight issues.

You've learnt that exercise plays a role too, particularly in maintaining weight once it has been lost. I hope you've learnt some strategies you can apply if you hate exercise.

You may need help to achieve what you want – joining a group, using an app, trying a therapy – but some people do succeed all on their own.

There are some simple hacks that can help you. These are the place to start if you are feeling overwhelmed. Remember the ones about the variety effect (Hack 08) or drinking water before a meal (Hack 58)? Get some small successes under your (loosening) belt!

Maybe your weight is part of a bigger picture – your lack of time for yourself or that small negative voice in your head. It's not just about your weight but about all aspects of your life.

If you feel you need a completely new approach, take a look at the stress in your life or your relationship with your parents. Notice that some hacks tell you that rather than focussing on restricting what you eat, you need to focus on feeling that you are a person in control of things. Once you feel more in control generally, you can control what you eat with less stress.

Remember also that fat shaming yourself or anyone else isn't helpful. Maybe you need to show the research to someone close to you, who is trying unsuccessfully to help you by criticising your weight and eating habits.

I hope you're as excited as I am about all the possibilities. Start today (not next Monday) and find new ways back to your true self.

Books by Jane Thurnell-Read

I'd appreciate it if you took the time to leave a review wherever you bought this book. Reviews help readers see books that would be a good fit for them. They also help me to sell more books.

All books are available on Amazon as eBooks and paperbacks. The first three are also available as audiobooks, via Amazon, Audible and iTunes.

- 190 Weight Loss Hacks: How to lose weight naturally and permanently without stress

- Menopause Weight Loss: Live well, sleep well, stop hot flashes and lose weight

- The Science of Healthy Ageing: Unlocking the Secrets to Longevity, Vitality, and Disease Prevention

Specialist books for CAM therapists

- Energy Mismatch for Kinesiologists, Dowsers & EAV Practitioners

- Verbal Questioning Skills for Kinesiologists & Dowsers

Jane's YouTube Channel

Lots of practical advice, insights, and straight-forward explanations about the latest research in health and wellbeing.

Do you want to eat better without getting stressed or annoying those you live with?

Do you want to sleep better? Maybe you have problems getting to sleep or staying asleep. Learn simple techniques you probably don't know already.

Are you wondering if you're too old to exercise? Get the answer explained in clear and accessible ways.

Learn about the latest menopause research. For example, does HRT increase your chances of getting dementia?

Understand why you shouldn't put bananas and berries together.

Do you know how many steps you need to take to benefit your health? (It's not 10,000!)

Do you want strategies to help you lose weight or strategies to maintain the weight you've already lost? We've got those too!

I also interview people who've changed their diets and found massive health benefits.

Check out my YouTube Channel for all this and more: @thrivingjane

Please review this book

I hope you have enjoyed reading this book.

Did you buy this book from Amazon? If you have found it useful, please take the time to review it on Amazon. It's so easy and quick:

Go to the Amazon page for this book

Scroll down to see the reviews.

Look for the button "Write a customer review" and click on that.

The more reviews there are for this book, the more likely Amazon is to show my book to prospective readers. You will be helping other people as well as me.

Thank you.

About the author

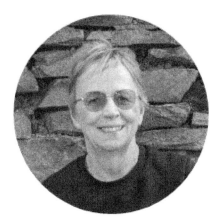

I have been a university lecturer, a complementary therapist and an entrepreneur over the years. But throughout that time, I've loved books and writing. I enjoy sharing difficult information and ideas with others in a way that doesn't dumb it down or disrespect people. People say that's one of my superpowers!

I'm now in my seventies – I'm fit, strong and healthy. That didn't happen by accident. In my twenties, I drank heavily (a quarter of a bottle of whisky a day) and smoked around 40 cigarettes a day. My diet consisted of toast, chocolate and orange juice. I learnt bit by bit how to change that and become happier and healthier.

In my late forties, I learnt to ride a bike. In my sixties, I fell in love with lifting heavy weights in the gym.

I know that small changes can have a big impact on our lives. I believe in sharing practical, research-based information that you can easily apply in your life too.

I want to inspire and inform you, so you can be happier and healthier than you've ever been.

You can connect with me on

Youtube: https://tinyurl.com/yt999-jtr

Instagram @thrivingjane

Website www.janethurnellread.com

1. https://hbr.org/2016/11/have-we-been-thinking-about-willpower-the-wrong-way-for-30-years

2. https://www.researchgate.net/publication/347315439_Morning_resolutions_evening_disillusions_Theories_of_willpower_affect_how_health_behaviours_change_across_the_day

3. https://www.sciencedaily.com/releases/2009/09/090924141749.htm

4. http://europepmc.org/article/MED/34149507

5. https://www.npr.org/2010/12/10/131967496/Thinking-About-Eating-May-Mean-Eating-Less

6. https://pubmed.ncbi.nlm.nih.gov/3612492/

7. https://www.sciencedaily.com/releases/2010/10/101018163110.htm

8. http://www.brianwansink.com/home/using-the-half-plate-rule

9. https://www.sciencedaily.com/releases/2010/01/100112085516.htm

10. https://www.verywellfit.com/what-does-halt-stand-for-4160620

11. https://www.hhhealth.com/2016/11/09/halt-a-tool-to-curb-emotional-eating/

12. https://theconversation.com/how-not-to-overeat-this-christmas-according-to-science-128709

13. https://pubmed.ncbi.nlm.nih.gov/25903253/

14. https://www.hriuk.org/health/your-health/nutrition/10-ways-to-combat-boredom-eating

15. https://www.ucl.ac.uk/school-life-medical-sciences/news/2019/feb/making-goals-public-could-hinder-weight-loss

16. https://www.inc.com/melissa-chu/announcing-your-goals-makes-you-less-likely
    -to-ach.html

17. https://www.hri.org.au/health/your-health/nutrition/10-healthy-food-hacks-for
    -summer

18. https://www.eurekalert.org/news-releases/564689

19. https://www.nih.gov/news-events/nih-research-matters/artificial-light-during-sle
    ep-linked-obesity

20. https://www.nhs.uk/live-well/healthy-weight/managing-your-weight/12-tips-to
    -help-you-lose-weight/

21. https://www.apa.org/topics/obesity/weight-control

22. https://www.bhf.org.uk/informationsupport/heart-matters-magazine/nutrition
    /ask-the-expert/when-to-eat-meals

23. https://www.sciencedaily.com/releases/2020/02/200219092539.htm

24. https://www.mayoclinic.org/healthy-lifestyle/weight-loss/expert-answers/food-a
    nd-nutrition/faq-20058449

25. https://www.forbes.com/health/body/the-pulse-with-dr-melina/

26. https://www.hsph.harvard.edu/nutritionsource/snacking/

27. https://www.hriuk.org/health/nutrition/10-healthy-eating-habits-to-get-into

28. https://www.menshealth.com/nutrition/g19546423/snacks-making-you-hungri
    er/

29. https://www.sleepfoundation.org/physical-health/weight-loss-and-sleep

30. https://www.ncbi.nlm.nih.gov/pmc/articles/PMC3763921/

31. https://news.byu.edu/intellect/teens-not-getting-enough-sleep-may-consume-4
    -5-extra-pounds-of-sugar-during-a-school-year-says-byu-research

32. https://www.headspace.com/

33. https://pubmed.ncbi.nlm.nih.gov/24720812/

34. https://www.ncbi.nlm.nih.gov/pmc/articles/PMC4505755/

35. https://sleep.biomedcentral.com/articles/10.1186/s41606-020-00047-x

36. https://pubmed.ncbi.nlm.nih.gov/33383648/

37. https://academic.oup.com/ajcn/article/113/1/154/5918527

38. https://www.sciencedaily.com/releases/2013/04/130430110321.htm

39. https://www.upi.com/Health_News/2013/05/11/Circadian-rhythm-ups-cravings-for-sweet-starchy-salty-snacks/63551368329101/?spt=su

40. https://www.eatright.org/health/wellness/healthy-habits/5-tips-to-curb-your-late-night-snacking

41. https://wexnermedical.osu.edu/blog/how-to-lose-weight-without-tanking-your-metabolism

42. https://www.sciencedaily.com/releases/2022/01/220112105657.htm

43. https://www.sciencedaily.com/releases/2013/09/130905113711.htm

44. https://www.retailwire.com/discussion/study-self-checkout-curtails-impulse-buys/

45. https://www.monash.edu/news/articles/5939

46. https://pubmed.ncbi.nlm.nih.gov/25959448/

47. https://www.sciencedaily.com/releases/2015/07/150707134212.htm

48. http://www.brianwansink.com/grocery-shoppers.html

49. http://www.brianwansink.com/grocery-shoppers.html

50. https://www.sciencedaily.com/releases/2019/05/190506080836.htm

51. https://www.liebertpub.com/doi/full/10.1089/acm.2020.0305

52. https://news.cornell.edu/stories/2006/02/candy-desk-candy-mouth-study-finds

53. https://www.ncbi.nlm.nih.gov/labs/pmc/articles/PMC3257626/

54. https://www.ncbi.nlm.nih.gov/labs/pmc/articles/PMC4646500/

55. https://www.nmcd-journal.com/article/S0939-4753(16)30329-5/fulltext

56. https://www.theguardian.com/environment/2022/jan/18/mind-boggling-hidden-cost-ecosystems-obsession-with-fish-oil-pills

57. https://www.nothingfishy.co/

58. https://clinmedjournals.org/articles/iaarm/international-archives-of-addiction-research-and-medicine-iaarm-1-010.pdf

59. https://news.illinois.edu/view/6367/240046

60. https://www.ncbi.nlm.nih.gov/labs/pmc/articles/PMC3772345/

61. https://news.umanitoba.ca/artificial-sweeteners-linked-to-risk-of-long-term-weight-gain-heart-disease-and-other-health-issues/

62. https://www.frontiersin.org/articles/10.3389/fnut.2020.598340/full

63. https://www.ncbi.nlm.nih.gov/labs/pmc/articles/PMC5912158/

64. https://www.cdc.gov/healthyweight/losing_weight/getting_started.html

65. https://www.healthcareevolve.ca/the-brain-and-obesity-part-6/

66. https://www.psychologytoday.com/gb/blog/fixing-families/201712/how-break-bad-habits

67. https://academic.oup.com/ajcn/article/114/6/1873/6369073

68. https://glycemicindex.com/

69. https://www.hsph.harvard.edu/nutritionsource/carbohydrates/carbohydrates-and-blood-sugar/

70. https://academic.oup.com/ajcn/article/98/3/641/4577039

71. http://www.futureme.org/

72. https://www.cdc.gov/healthyweight/losing_weight/getting_started.html

73. https://www.sciencedirect.com/science/article/pii/B9780128026908000062

74. https://www.healthcareevolve.ca/plotting-your-weight-loss-journey-with-values-instead-of-goals/

75. https://theconversation.com/chronic-stress-could-be-making-you-fat-71958

76. https://www.nhs.uk/mental-health/self-help/guides-tools-and-activities/tips-to-reduce-stress/

77. https://www.mindbodygreen.com/0-8370/15-affirmations-that-will-help-you-lose-weight.html

78. https://www.sciencedirect.com/science/article/pii/B9780128026908000062

79. https://www.healthcareevolve.ca/plotting-your-weight-loss-journey-with-values-instead-of-goals/

80. https://www.heart.org/en/healthy-living/healthy-eating/losing-weight

81. https://academic.oup.com/jcem/article/97/7/A33/2833215

82. https://www.sydney.edu.au/news-opinion/news/2019/02/21/the-new-exercise-trend-that-s-made-for-everyone.html

83. https://theconversation.com/resistance-training-heres-why-its-so-effective-for-weight-loss-146453

84. https://www.pbrc.edu/news/media/2021/metabolism-milestones.aspx

85. https://www.health.harvard.edu/healthbeat/is-hefty-the-new-healthy

86. https://theconversation.com/ten-habits-of-people-who-lose-weight-and-keep-it-off-101387

87. https://www.headspace.com/

88. https://www.sciencedirect.com/science/article/abs/pii/S019566631000365X

89. https://www.liebertpub.com/doi/10.1089/act.2018.29182.lnl

90. https://www.mcgill.ca/newsroom/channels/news/mindfulness-training-shows-promise-maintaining-weight-loss-283028

91. https://www.bda.uk.com/resource/mindful-eating.html

92. https://ggia.berkeley.edu/practice/raisin_meditation

93. https://mbsrtraining.com/mindfulness-exercises-by-jon-kabat-zinn/mindfully-eating-a-raisin-script/

94. https://www.evelyntribole.com/what-is-intuitive-eating/

95. https://www.intuitiveeating.org/

96. https://academic.oup.com/ajcn/article/110/1/10/5510580?searchresult=1

97. http://www.brianwansink.com/qa-blogus/what-is-the-mindless-margin

98. https://www.mayoclinic.org/healthy-lifestyle/weight-loss/expert-answers/fast-weight-loss/faq-20058289

99. https://pubmed.ncbi.nlm.nih.gov/19661958/

100. https://onlinelibrary.wiley.com/doi/10.1002/oby.21167

101. https://thehealthsciencesacademy.org/health-tips/water-for-weight-loss/

102. https://hub.jhu.edu/at-work/2020/01/15/focus-on-wellness-drinking-more-wat er/

103. http://pwlclincoln.com/the-link-between-dehydration-and-metabolism/

104. https://www.ncbi.nlm.nih.gov/labs/pmc/articles/PMC3809630/

105. https://www.hriuk.org/health/your-health/nutrition/10-ways-to-combat-bored om-eating

106. https://theconversation.com/why-frequent-dieting-makes-you-put-on-weight-a nd-what-to-do-about-it-69329

107. https://www.mayoclinic.org/healthy-lifestyle/weight-loss/expert-answers/fast-w eight-loss/faq-20058289

108. https://pubmed.ncbi.nlm.nih.gov/25459211/

109. https://www.ncbi.nlm.nih.gov/labs/pmc/articles/PMC5702468/

110. https://theconversation.com/microbiome-good-gut-bacteria-really-could-help-y ou-lose-weight-new-study-168036

111. https://atlasbiomed.com/blog/link-between-gut-bacteria-and-weight-loss/

112. https://www.bbc.co.uk/food/articles/plantbased_weightloss?

113. https://atlasbiomed.com/blog/link-between-gut-bacteria-and-weight-loss/

114. https://veganuary.com/veganism-weight-loss/

115. https://atlasbiomed.com/blog/link-between-gut-bacteria-and-weight-loss/

116. https://health.clevelandclinic.org/why-are-certain-foods-so-addictive/

117. https://www.ncbi.nlm.nih.gov/labs/pmc/articles/PMC4150387/

118. https://www.ncbi.nlm.nih.gov/labs/pmc/articles/PMC5912158/

119. https://www.scientificamerican.com/article/how-sugar-and-fat-trick-the-brain-into-wanting-more-food/

120. https://www.scientificamerican.com/article/how-sugar-and-fat-trick-the-brain-into-wanting-more-food/

121. https://news.uchicago.edu/story/trying-protect-teens-against-junk-food-marketing-tap-their-desire-rebel

122. https://well.blogs.nytimes.com/2015/08/09/coca-cola-funds-scientists-who-shift-blame-for-obesity-away-from-bad-diets

123. https://theconversation.com/is-it-our-fault-if-we-eat-too-many-calories-63730

124. https://theconversation.com/dieting-may-slow-metabolism-but-it-doesnt-ruin-it-154620

125. https://www.racmn.com/blog/consider-metabolic-adaptation-for-more-effective-dieting

126. https://onlinelibrary.wiley.com/doi/full/10.1002/oby.21538

127. https://theconversation.com/dieting-may-slow-metabolism-but-it-doesnt-ruin-it-154620

128. https://www.mayoclinic.org/healthy-lifestyle/weight-loss/in-depth/weight-loss-plateau/art-20044615

129. https://www.sydney.edu.au/news-opinion/news/2017/10/05/7-ways-to-tackle-obesity-.html

130. https://www.sydney.edu.au/medicine-health/news-and-events/2020/03/23/how-to-prevent-weight-regain.html

131. https://www.racmn.com/blog/consider-metabolic-adaptation-for-more-effective-dieting

132. https://pubmed.ncbi.nlm.nih.gov/10643690/

133. https://www.apa.org/science/about/psa/2018/05/calorie-deprivation

134. https://news.cuanschutz.edu/news-stories/cu-anschutz-study-reveals-exercise-is-more-critical-than-diet-to-maintain-weight-loss

135. https://theconversation.com/dieting-may-slow-metabolism-but-it-doesnt-ruin-it-154620

136. https://www.cdc.gov/physicalactivity/basics/pa-health/

137. https://pubmed.ncbi.nlm.nih.gov/16854220/

138. http://www.nwcr.ws/Research/default.htm

139. https://pubmed.ncbi.nlm.nih.gov/24355667/

140. https://source.wustl.edu/2017/12/six-tips-adopting-healthy-behaviors/

141. https://pubmed.ncbi.nlm.nih.gov/10224727/

142. https://pubmed.ncbi.nlm.nih.gov/11011910/

143. https://www.liebertpub.com/doi/10.1089/act.2017.29116.jha

144. https://www.health.harvard.edu/blog/why-keep-a-food-diary-2019013115855

145. https://www.tops.org/tops/tops/TOPS/FeaturedArticles/FocusOnYou/emotional-eating.aspx

146. https://www.apa.org/topics/obesity/weight-gain

147. https://today.duke.edu/2019/02/tracking-food-leads-losing-pounds

148. https://jech.bmj.com/content/74/3/269

149. https://www.lboro.ac.uk/media-centre/press-releases/2019/december/labelling-foods-amount-of-physical-activity-needed/

150. https://www.onhealth.com/content/1/calories_burned_during_fitness

151. https://www.sciencedirect.com/science/article/pii/S1756464621000980

152. https://www.sciencedaily.com/releases/2020/05/200521115627.htm

153. https://www.sciencedirect.com/science/article/pii/S235215461500131X

154. https://pubmed.ncbi.nlm.nih.gov/18589027/

155. https://www.sciencedaily.com/releases/2009/11/091104085230.htm

156. https://www.sydney.edu.au/news-opinion/news/2020/01/21/6-steps-to-success ful-weight-loss-for-women.html

157. https://pressroom.usc.edu/habit-makes-bad-food-too-easy-to-swallow/

158. https://www.heart.org/en/healthy-living/healthy-eating/eat-smart/nutrition-basi cs/portion-size-versus-serving-size

159. https://www.heart.org/en/healthy-living/healthy-eating/eat-smart/nutrition-basi cs/portion-size-versus-serving-size

160. https://www.nhlbi.nih.gov/health/educational/lose_wt/behavior.htm

161. https://www.ncbi.nlm.nih.gov/pmc/articles/PMC4337741/

162. https://blogs.biomedcentral.com/on-health/2019/10/29/can-smaller-plates-help -us-to-eat-less/

163. https://pubmed.ncbi.nlm.nih.gov/24341317/

164. https://theconversation.com/playing-with-the-senses-can-change-how-food-tast es-75468

165. https://pubmed.ncbi.nlm.nih.gov/24005858/

166. https://news.illinois.edu/view/6367/204477

167. https://www.apa.org/topics/obesity/mind-body-health

168. https://www.amdietetics.com/articles/coping-with-lapses-when-trying-to-lose-weight

169. https://link.springer.com/article/10.1007/s13668-020-00326-0

170. https://www.ncbi.nlm.nih.gov/labs/pmc/articles/PMC6186388/

171. https://www.heart.org/en/healthy-living/healthy-eating/losing-weight/conquer-cravings-with-these-healthy-substitutions

172. https://pubmed.ncbi.nlm.nih.gov/20025372/

173. https://www.choosehelp.com/topics/recovery/cravings-mindfulness-urge-surfing

174. https://www.medicinenet.com/script/main/art.asp?articlekey=154184

175. https://www.ncbi.nlm.nih.gov/labs/pmc/articles/PMC5507106/

176. https://www.ahajournals.org/doi/10.1161/CIRCRESAHA.119.315896

177. https://www.hsph.harvard.edu/obesity-prevention-source/obesity-consequences/health-effects/

178. https://www.psychologytoday.com/us/blog/nourish/201010/my-bold-new-plan-the-sit-down-diet

179. https://www.hriuk.org/health/your-health/nutrition/10-ways-to-combat-boredom-eating

180. https://www.mindbodygreen.com/0-8370/15-affirmations-that-will-help-you-lose-weight.html

181. https://www.eatright.org/health/wellness/fad-diets/negative-calorie-foods-still-count

182. https://blog.thecenterformindfuleating.org/2021/10/how-do-i-know-i-am-hungry-exploring.html

183. https://www.helpguide.org/articles/diets/emotional-eating.htm

184. https://today.uic.edu/research-review-shows-intermittent-fasting-works-for-weight-loss-health-changes

185. https://academic.oup.com/ajcn/article/108/5/933/5201451

186. https://www.surrey.ac.uk/news/changes-breakfast-and-dinner-timings-can-reduce-body-fat

187. https://www.forbes.com/health/body/the-pulse-with-dr-melina/

188. https://www.liebertpub.com/doi/10.1089/act.2021.29319.klu

189. https://www.npr.org/sections/thetwo-way/2016/09/13/493739074/50-years-ago-sugar-industry-quietly-paid-scientists-to-point-blame-at-fat

190. https://theconversation.com/sugar-detox-cutting-carbs-a-doctor-explains-why-you-should-keep-fruit-on-the-menu-173992

191. https://theconversation.com/sugar-detox-cutting-carbs-a-doctor-explains-why-you-should-keep-fruit-on-the-menu-173992

192. https://theconversation.com/keto-diet-a-dietitian-on-what-you-need-to-know-99867

193. https://theconversation.com/do-low-carb-diets-help-you-lose-weight-heres-what-the-science-says-176368

194. https://theconversation.com/sugar-detox-cutting-carbs-a-doctor-explains-why-you-should-keep-fruit-on-the-menu-173992

195. https://www.hsph.harvard.edu/nutritionsource/healthy-weight/diet-reviews/ketogenic-diet/

196. https://www.hriuk.org/health/nutrition/going-low-carb

197. https://www.hsph.harvard.edu/nutritionsource/carbohydrates/

198. https://theconversation.com/do-low-carb-diets-help-you-lose-weight-heres-what-the-science-says-176368

199. https://www.hsph.harvard.edu/nutritionsource/healthy-weight/healthy-dietary-styles/

200. https://pubmed.ncbi.nlm.nih.gov/12566139/

201. https://www.health.harvard.edu/blog/theres-no-sugar-coating-it-all-calories-are-not-created-equal-2016110410602

202. https://www.forbes.com/health/body/the-pulse-with-dr-melina/

203. https://nutrition.bmj.com/content/early/2019/08/27/bmjnph-2019-000034

204. https://www.sciencedaily.com/releases/2017/09/170920100107.htm

205. https://theconversation.com/beach-body-row-misses-the-key-points-about-protein-and-weight-loss-40997

206. https://www.ncbi.nlm.nih.gov/labs/pmc/articles/PMC7539343/

207. https://source.wustl.edu/2016/10/high-protein-diet-curbs-metabolic-benefits-weight-loss/

208. https://www.ncbi.nlm.nih.gov/labs/pmc/articles/PMC6768815/

209. https://www.acpjournals.org/doi/10.7326/M14-0611?articleid=2118594

210. https://www.nutrition.org.uk/healthyliving/basics/fibre.html

211. https://www.health.harvard.edu/staying-healthy/how-to-get-more-fiber-in-your-diet

212. https://www.zest-health.com/blog/15-ways-with-pulses

213. https://ods.od.nih.gov/factsheets/WeightLoss-Consumer/

214. https://www.mcgill.ca/oss/article/weight-loss/konjac-and-weight-loss

215. https://www.sydney.edu.au/news-opinion/news/2018/09/12/3-reasons-you-nev er-have-to-diet-again.html

216. https://www.ncbi.nlm.nih.gov/labs/pmc/articles/PMC6330473/

217. https://pubmed.ncbi.nlm.nih.gov/14647183/

218. https://www.ncbi.nlm.nih.gov/pmc/articles/PMC3740215/

219. https://theconversation.com/metabolic-confusion-diet-wont-boost-metabolism -but-it-could-have-other-benefits-150341

220. https://www.hsph.harvard.edu/nutritionsource/healthy-weight/diet-reviews/pal eo-diet/

221. https://www.hsph.harvard.edu/nutritionsource/healthy-weight/diet-reviews/pal eo-diet/

222. https://www.sciencedaily.com/releases/2019/07/190722105935.htm

223. https://www.sciencedaily.com/releases/2016/02/160218114753.htm

224. https://pubmed.ncbi.nlm.nih.gov/11883916/

225. https://www.mayoclinic.org/healthy-lifestyle/weight-loss/in-depth/weight-loss/ art-20048466

226. https://theconversation.com/calories-or-macros-nutritionist-explains-which-wor ks-best-for-weight-loss-or-building-muscle-141096

227. https://www.mayoclinic.org/healthy-lifestyle/weight-loss/in-depth/weight-loss/ art-20048466

228. https://www.niddk.nih.gov/health-information/weight-management/myths-nut rition-physical-activity

229. https://www.wholelifechallenge.com/why-you-need-to-put-yourself-first-and-ho w-to-do-it/

230. https://www.hopkinsmedicine.org/health/wellness-and-prevention/bloating-causes-and-prevention-tips

231. https://www.hindawi.com/journals/isrn/2012/721820/

232. https://www.amdietetics.com/articles/beating-the-bloat-have-you-considered-stress

233. https://www.health.harvard.edu/diseases-and-conditions/the-gut-brain-connection

234. https://www.amdietetics.com/articles/beating-the-bloat-have-you-considered-stress

235. https://news.illinois.edu/view/6367/907033287

236. https://www.sciencedaily.com/releases/2020/12/201215175758.htm

237. https://www.ncbi.nlm.nih.gov/labs/pmc/articles/PMC5111772/#jhn12390-bib-0009

238. https://theconversation.com/three-ways-behavioural-psychology-might-help-you-lose-weight-156257

239. https://www.sciencedaily.com/releases/2007/09/070914190944.htm

240. https://academic.oup.com/her/article/22/4/532/633956

241. https://www.nhlbi.nih.gov/health/educational/lose_wt/behavior.htm

242. https://www.bda.uk.com/resource/weight-loss.html

243. https://blog.thecenterformindfuleating.org/2021/11/understanding-relationship-with-food.html

244. https://www.apa.org/topics/obesity/mind-body-health

245. https://www.liebertpub.com/doi/full/10.1089/acm.2020.0104

246. https://www.sciencedirect.com/science/article/abs/pii/S2095496420301229#!

247. https://www.mayoclinic.org/healthy-lifestyle/weight-loss/expert-answers/weight-loss-hypnosis/faq-20058291

248. https://iaap-journals.onlinelibrary.wiley.com/doi/10.1111/aphw.12070

249. https://petastapleton.com/

250. https://www.nhs.uk/mental-health/talking-therapies-medicine-treatments/talking-therapies-and-counselling/cognitive-behavioural-therapy-cbt/overview/

251. https://www.mcgill.ca/newsroom/channels/news/habit-change-key-success-weight-loss-290145

252. https://www.myfitnesspal.com/

253. https://www.myfitnesspal.com/

254. https://www.sciencedaily.com/releases/2008/12/081215074404.htm

255. https://www.psychotherapynetworker.org/blog/details/615/a-cognitive-behavioral-therapy-solution-for-losing

256. https://www.ncbi.nlm.nih.gov/labs/pmc/articles/PMC6022277/

257. https://pmj.bmj.com/content/96/1134/221

258. https://www.ncbi.nlm.nih.gov/labs/pmc/articles/PMC4877795/

259. https://journals.lww.com/md-journal/fulltext/2019/06280/auricular_acupressure_for_overweight_and_obese.51.aspx

260. https://mhealth.jmir.org/2019/5/e14386/

261. https://pubmed.ncbi.nlm.nih.gov/25183702/

262. https://www.ncbi.nlm.nih.gov/labs/pmc/articles/PMC6446167/

263. https://pubmed.ncbi.nlm.nih.gov/35054828/

264. https://pubmed.ncbi.nlm.nih.gov/33186794/

265. https://pubmed.ncbi.nlm.nih.gov/18433791/

266. https://www.nccih.nih.gov/research/research-results/study-sees-beneficial-role-of-yoga-in-weight-loss-program-for-adults-with-obesity-or-overweight

267. https://www.ncbi.nlm.nih.gov/labs/pmc/articles/PMC4995338/

268. https://www.apa.org/monitor/jan04/teaming

269. https://www.ucl.ac.uk/ioe/news/2016/oct/support-group-leaders-and-peers-crucial-successful-weight-loss

270. https://www.apa.org/monitor/jan04/teaming

271. https://drexel.edu/now/archive/2020/December/Sharing-Health-Data-to-Maintain-Weight-Loss/

272. http://www.nwcr.ws/people/default.htm

273. https://news.illinois.edu/view/6367/204477

274. https://source.wustl.edu/2017/12/six-tips-adopting-healthy-behaviors/

275. https://www.sciencedaily.com/releases/2021/11/211122135407.htm

276. https://www.sciencedaily.com/releases/2020/08/200827101837.htm

277. https://www.12step.com/articles/12-step-lifestyle/12-step-program-weight-loss

278. https://www.foodaddicts.org/

279. https://oa.org/

280. https://en.wikipedia.org/wiki/Overeaters_Anonymous

281. https://en.wikipedia.org/wiki/Food_Addicts_in_Recovery_Anonymous

282. https://www.hindawi.com/journals/jobe/2015/763680/

283. https://pubmed.ncbi.nlm.nih.gov/26896865/

284. https://pubmed.ncbi.nlm.nih.gov/18976879/

285. https://ijbnpa.biomedcentral.com/articles/10.1186/s12966-015-0267-4

286. https://www.ncbi.nlm.nih.gov/labs/pmc/articles/PMC8277333/

287. https://www.nhlbi.nih.gov/health/educational/lose_wt/behavior.htm

288. https://onlinelibrary.wiley.com/doi/10.1111/obr.12816

289. https://www.ncbi.nlm.nih.gov/labs/pmc/articles/PMC6327254/

290. https://www.unm.edu/~lkravitz/Article folder/Mealreplacement.html

291. https://www.phc.ox.ac.uk/news/blog/eight-myths-about-meal-replacement-diets-debunked

292. https://alcoholchange.org.uk/alcohol-facts/fact-sheets/alcohol-and-calories

293. https://alcoholchange.org.uk/alcohol-facts/fact-sheets/alcohol-and-calories

294. https://theconversation.com/two-glasses-of-wine-might-add-more-sugar-to-your-diet-than-eating-a-doughnut-177301

295. https://www.hriuk.org/health/nutrition/10-healthy-eating-habits-to-get-into

296. https://www.nidirect.gov.uk/articles/what-happens-when-you-drink-alcohol

297. https://www.alcohol.org/effects/inhibitions/

298. https://www.ncbi.nlm.nih.gov/labs/pmc/articles/PMC6565398/

299. https://www.nationaleatingdisorders.org/learn/general-information/ten-steps

300. https://theconversation.com/how-being-in-nature-makes-us-appreciate-our-bodies-and-reject-unrealistic-beauty-standards-63145

301. https://news.ok.ubc.ca/2017/06/14/want-to-feel-stronger-and-thinner-get-some-exercise/

302. https://clinicaltrials.gov/

303. https://beta.clinicaltrials.gov/

304. https://greatergood.berkeley.edu/article/item/the_cost_of_blaming_parents

305. https://www.sciencedaily.com/releases/2019/09/190917133050.htm

306. https://www.facebook.com/watch/?v=215713596824302

307. https://theconversation.com/understanding-body-signals-could-be-a-key-factor-in-eating-disorders-111559

308. https://onlinelibrary.wiley.com/doi/10.1002/oby.20976

309. https://www.shape.com/healthy-eating/diet-tips/10-food-pushers-and-how-respond

310. https://www.sciencedaily.com/releases/2014/10/141014114118.htm

311. https://www.sciencedaily.com/releases/2010/03/100322171024.htm

312. https://www.journals.uchicago.edu/doi/full/10.1086/710251

313. https://www.sussex.ac.uk/broadcast/read/52535

314. https://academic.oup.com/ajcn/article/97/4/728/4577025?login=true

315. https://www.lboro.ac.uk/service/publicity/news-releases/2011/110_diet.html

316. https://www.wcrf.org/can-too-much-screen-time-affect-our-weight/

317. https://www.wcrf.org/dietandcancer/body-fatness-and-weight-gain/

318. https://onlinelibrary.wiley.com/doi/10.1038/oby.2006.209

319. https://theconversation.com/the-best-way-to-ditch-bad-habits-what-science-can-teach-us-128724

320. https://www.michaeldpollock.com/mindset-motivation-perseverance/

321. https://theconversation.com/five-rules-from-psychology-to-help-keep-your-new-years-resolutions-128816

322. https://www.researchgate.net/publication/315422561_Vice_and_Virtue_Food_Perceived_Impulsiveness_and_Healthfulness_of_100_Food_Items

323. https://jamanetwork.com/journals/jamapsychiatry/fullarticle/210608

324. https://www.apa.org/topics/obesity/mind-body-health

325. https://www.sciencefocus.com/science/is-hot-food-more-filling-than-cold-food/

326. https://academic.oup.com/jcr/article-abstract/47/4/523/5815985

327. https://www.sciencedaily.com/releases/2013/04/130409131215.htm

328. https://pubmed.ncbi.nlm.nih.gov/9697946/

329. https://www.sciencedaily.com/releases/2019/05/190523091305.htm

330. https://www.jandonline.org/article/S2212-2672(13)01415-9/fulltext

331. https://www.bmj.com/content/363/bmj.k4867

332. https://theconversation.com/why-now-is-the-best-time-to-go-on-a-diet-or-the-science-of-post-holiday-weight-loss-52075

333. https://santiago-compostela.net/

334. https://matadornetwork.com/read/amazing-pilgrimage-paths/

335. https://www.nationaleatingdisorders.org/blog/tips-surviving-thanksgiving-recovery

336. https://nutritionj.biomedcentral.com/articles/10.1186/1475-2891-10-9

337. https://www.hsph.harvard.edu/obesity-prevention-source/obesity-causes/genes-and-obesity/

338. https://www.ncbi.nlm.nih.gov/pmc/articles/PMC6736184/

339. https://www.sciencedaily.com/releases/2012/03/120314142833.htm

340. https://www.ncl.ac.uk/press/articles/archive/2016/09/geneandweightloss/

341. https://www.hsph.harvard.edu/obesity-prevention-source/obesity-causes/genes-and-obesity/

342. https://www.mayoclinic.org/healthy-lifestyle/weight-loss/expert-answers/caffeine/faq-20058459

343. https://consumer.healthday.com/vitamins-and-nutrition-information-27/caffeine-health-news-89/could-your-morning-coffee-be-a-weight-loss-tool-753803.html

344. https://www.sciencedaily.com/releases/2020/10/201002091053.htm

345. https://nutritionj.biomedcentral.com/articles/10.1186/1475-2891-10-9

346. https://www.psychologytoday.com/gb/blog/fixing-families/201712/how-break-bad-habits

347. https://www.sydney.edu.au/news-opinion/news/2016/02/11/experts-rank-the-best-apps-for-weight-loss.html

348. https://www.noom.com/

349. https://www.ncbi.nlm.nih.gov/labs/pmc/articles/PMC7326765/

350. https://www.jmir.org/2021/4/e25160/

351. https://pubmed.ncbi.nlm.nih.gov/15976148/

352. https://pubmed.ncbi.nlm.nih.gov/21289225/

353. https://www.ncbi.nlm.nih.gov/labs/pmc/articles/PMC2128765/

354. https://pubmed.ncbi.nlm.nih.gov/15389416/

355. https://www.cdc.gov/

356. https://www.instagram.com/thrivingjane/

357. https://www.amdietetics.com/articles/5-easy-ways-to-increase-your-vegetable-in take

358. https://www.hriuk.org/health/nutrition/setting-up-healthy-habits-for-success

359. https://www.ncbi.nlm.nih.gov/pmc/articles/PMC7399879/

360. https://www.ncbi.nlm.nih.gov/labs/pmc/articles/PMC4025876/

361. https://www.cambridgenetwork.co.uk/node/469697

362. https://www.nhs.uk/conditions/weight-loss-surgery/

363. https://www.ncbi.nlm.nih.gov/labs/pmc/articles/PMC5523816/

364. https://www.sciencedaily.com/releases/2020/08/200812094902.htm

365. https://pubmed.ncbi.nlm.nih.gov/32091656/

366. https://www.plymouth.ac.uk/news/weight-loss-can-be-boosted-fivefold-thanks -to-novel-mental-imagery-technique-research-shows

367. https://www.researchgate.net/publication/316230966_Do_images_of_a_persona lised_future_body_shape_help_with_weight_loss_A_randomised_controlled_st udy

368. https://www.sciencedaily.com/releases/2011/02/110225122818.htm

369. https://www.verywellfit.com/how-often-should-i-eat-3495751

370. https://academic.oup.com/jcem/article/97/7/A33/2833215

371. https://www.scientificamerican.com/article/need-more-self-control-try-a-simple-ritual/

372. https://www.acefitness.org/education-and-resources/lifestyle/blog/44/why-is-the-concept-of-spot-reduction-considered-a-myth/#about-pane

373. https://jamesclear.com/behavior-change-paradox

374. https://corporate-edge.com.au/ce-john/a-guide-to-getting-out-of-the-comfort-zone-trap/

375. https://www.hsph.harvard.edu/obesity-prevention-source/obesity-consequences/health-effects/

376. https://www.sciencedaily.com/releases/2020/11/201113124049.htm

Printed in Great Britain
by Amazon

44781587R00188